WATCHING TV IS NOT REQUIRED

This book was created over years of discussion, classroom experiments, exercises, and interaction. The book is also the process and product of the interaction of two individuals working with ideas. Its creation is the antithesis of what we are critiquing. It is the result of a dialogue and human relationship. The book addresses a very different relationship, a "relationship" to television ... a "televisionship," a one-dimensional imprinting relationship without dialogue or living human interaction. It examines a relationship with Plato's "cave" and the contemporary media matrix that continues its existence.

Bernard McGrane is a professor in the Sociology Department at Chapman University. He is the author of *Beyond Anthropology, Society and the Other*, *The Un-TV and the 10 MPH Car: Exploriments in Personal Freedom and Everyday Life*, *This Book is Not Required, An Emotional Survival Manual for Students*, and he is also featured in two educational videos: *The Ad and the Id: Sex, Death and Subliminal Advertising* and *The Ad and the Ego: Advertising and Identity*.

John Gunderson teaches at Dana Hills High School and Chapman University. His work focuses on the belief education can transform lives through passionate teaching grounded in theory and philosophy. He actively publishes work on diverse topics including: teaching and learning, school reform, college life, and the media.

Contemporary Sociological Perspectives

Edited by Valerie Jenness, University of California, Irvine and Jodi O'Brien, Seattle University

This innovative series is for all readers interested in books that provide frameworks for making sense of the complexities of contemporary social life. Each of the books in this series uses a sociological lens to provide current critical and analytical perspectives on significant social issues, patterns and trends. The series consists of books that integrate the best ideas in sociological thought with an aim toward public education and engagement. These books are designed for use in the classroom as well as for scholars and socially curious general readers.

Published:

Political Justice and Religious Values by Charles F. Andrain

GIS and Spatial Analysis for the Social Sciences by Robert Nash Parker and Emily K. Asencio

Hoop Dreams on Wheels: Disability and the Competitive Wheelchair Athlete by Ronald J. Berger

Forthcoming:

The Internet and Inequality by James C. Witte

Media and Middle Class Moms by Lara Descartes and Conrad Kottak

Sociology of Music by Michael B. MacDonald

Race, Justice and the New Genetics by Sandra Soo-Jin Lee

Intimate Impostors: The Social Psychology of Romantic Deception by Sally Caldwell

Regression Unplugged by Sally Caldwell and Robert Abbey

Violence Against Women by Douglas Brownridge

Gender Circuits by Eve Shapiro

WATCHING TV
IS NOT REQUIRED

Thinking About Media And
Thinking About Thinking

Bernard McGrane
John Gunderson

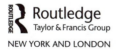

Routledge
Taylor & Francis Group

NEW YORK AND LONDON

First published 2010
by Routledge
270 Madison Ave, New York, NY 10016

Simultaneously published in the UK
by Routledge
2 Park Square, Milton Park, Abingdon, Oxon OX14 4RN

Routledge is an imprint of the Taylor & Francis Group, an informa business

Typeset in Caslon by HWA Text and Data Management, London
Printed and bound in the United States of America on acid-free paper by
Edwards Brothers, Inc.

Library of Congress Cataloging in Publication Data
McGrane, Bernard.
    Watching TV is not required : thinking about media and thinking about thinking /
Bernard McGrane, John Gunderson.
        p. cm. – (Contemporary sociological perspectives)
    1. Television—Social aspects. 2. Television—Psychological aspects. I. Gunderson,
John. II. Title.
    PN1992.6.M378 2009
    302.23´45–dc22   2009002607

ISBN10: 0–415–99486–1 (hbk)
ISBN10: 0–415–99487–X (pbk)

ISBN13: 978–0–415–99486–6 (hbk)
ISBN13: 978–0–415–99487–3 (pbk)

To my partner, my friend, my teacher, my love, Rupa

(Bernard McGrane)

To Jack and Dan, I'm proud to be your father. You are my eternal sunlight.

(John Gunderson)

Contents

Preface for Educators

The Dalai Lama of Tibet practices mediation four hours a day. The average American practices "television meditation" four hours a day. This book deals with the defining role of television in the experience of socialization, of identity and the occurrence of reality. Television is *not just television*. This book is an argument and an exploration based on the view that television has become internalized as our *third parent* and argues that the blending of TV and the parent category is deep and powerful. It also strives to uncover the *Matrix*-like social maintenance of media power through a variety of phenomenological and ethnomethodological exercises (for example, count the technical events that occur in a 10-minute sample of ordinary television); field projects (for example, visit a toy store as an anthropological field ethnographer after consciously watching a sample of ordinary children's television); together with mindfulness meditation techniques (for example, attentively watch an ordinary television set for a specified time without turning it on). These enterprises are all designed to de-hypnotize us from our ordinary media-matrix trance.

This book aspires to make students more consciously aware of and actively, perhaps urgently, curious about the influence the media has had on them by provoking them to re-look into their own, ordinary media experience. It invites them to playfully-yet-seriously engage with certain types of norm-breaching "experiments" on their all-too-familiar experiences of ordinary television in our media-driven culture. It is designed for a participatory curriculum rather than one grounded on the transmission and accumulation of information. The "exercises" or "experiments" are followed by "results" and "reports" that have occurred with our own students. All this is done within an ongoing critical sociological conversation and commentary on the role of contemporary media in our public and private life. For our readers, we recommend doing the exercises yourself *before* reading about them. For our fellow teachers, we recommend assigning them to your students with the obligation of doing some type of brief write-up about their own experiences *before* having them read about the experiences of others that are provided in the text. Using this strategy will help you to maintain a "beginners mind" and not have the experiences of others cloud or predetermine your insights and discoveries.

Much of the thrust of this work is not to engage in traditional media bashing but rather to engage in media awareness and media literacy: This awareness and literacy is vital for our survival and mental well-being in contemporary culture. The purpose of this supplementary text is to make available to a wide variety of media courses—in sociology, political science, psychology, and cultural studies—an engaging, demanding, confronting, highly personal inquiry into our *social relationship* to the media, especially television. Through a series of iconoclastic discussions and analyses and an accompanying series of powerful exercises, the text works *to un-conceal television as our third parent.* From a critical sociological framework with a unique emphasis on socialization theory, we call television our "third parent" to highlight its *enormous yet highly indeterminate influence on us.* The sociological challenge of this work is to reveal the presence and normative structure of the commercial media within the very heart of our personal, intimate experience of ourselves. The ongoing mantra or koan, "Where does television end and my self begin?" resonates through the entire text. The pedagogical challenge is, as it were, to get fish to become aware that they are swimming in water.

This work is grounded in two contemporary streams feeding into the overall discipline of modern sociology: ethnomethodology and Buddhist sociology. Ethnomethodology studies the social construction of reality. Its focus is the methods and ways that we ordinarily achieve the *experience of ordinariness* and of ordinary reality—how we skillfully and interactionally achieve this orderly ordinariness and simultaneously forget that we achieve it and rather take social reality to be given, substantial, external, and independent of ourselves. (The philosophical foundation of ethnomethodology rests on the working hypothesis that reality is what we say it is and collectively agree it to be—*including* saying and agreeing that it is autonomous, objective, and independent of what we say and agree.) Buddhist sociology studies the social construction of self-identity. In its meditative and mindfulness practice dimension, it engages its students in a series of structured personal practices, experiences, and experiments wherein they use themselves as sociological laboratories. These experiences often abruptly cut through our ordinary bedrock experience of identity/ego and allow for a paradigm shifting and radically new experience of ourselves and our ordinary, taken-for-granted identity. We have found these experiments to be wonderful instruments for personal growth and awareness. We have also found them to be powerful pedagogical strategies for opening a dialogue of spontaneous discovery with students that is engaging, penetrating, personal and deep.

Preview: The Parable of Plato's Cave

This book is not television. This book is about our *relationship* to television. Hence, we think it is strangely appropriate to begin 2500 years ago with an ancient Greek philosopher's parable about "television training and the human condition." In Book VII of Plato's *The Republic*, we hear Socrates describe to Glaucon our contemporary physical situation of watching a TV in a darkened living room or a film in a darkened movie theatre. His description simultaneously addresses the plots of the 1998 film, *The Truman Show*, and the 1999 film, *The Matrix*, and, of-course, the "parable of the cave":

> "Next then," I said, "take the following parable of education and ignorance as a picture of the condition of our nature. Imagine mankind as dwelling in an underground cave with a long entrance open to the light across the whole width of the cave; in this they have been from childhood, with necks and legs fettered, so they have to stay where they are. They cannot move their heads round because of the fetters, and they can only look forward, but light comes to them from fire burning behind them higher up at a distance. Between the fire and the prisoners is a road above their level, and along it imagine a low wall has been built, as puppet showmen have screens in front of their people over which they work their puppets."
>
> "I see," he said.
>
> "See, then, bearers carrying along this wall all sorts of articles which they hold projecting above the wall, statues of men and other living things, made of stone or wood and all kinds of stuff, some of the bearers speaking and some silent, as you might expect."

"What a remarkable image," he said, "and what remarkable prisoners!"

"Just like ourselves," I said. "For, first of all, tell me this: What do you think such people would have seen of themselves and each other except their shadows, which the fire cast on the opposite wall of the cave?"

"I don't see how they could see anything else," said he, "if they were compelled to keep their heads unmoving all their lives!"

"Very well, what of the things being carried along? Would not this be the same?"

"Of course it would."

"Suppose the prisoners were able to talk together, don't you think that when they named the shadows which they saw passing they would believe they were naming things?"

"Necessarily."

"Then if their prison had an echo from the opposite wall whenever one of the passing bearers uttered a sound, would they not suppose that the passing shadow must be making the sound? Don't you think so?"

"Indeed I do," he said.

"If so," said I, "such persons would certainly believe that there were no realities except those shadows of handmade things."

"So it must be," said he.

"Now consider," said I, "what their release would be like, and their cure from these fetters and their folly; let us imagine whether it might naturally be something like this. One might be released, and compelled suddenly to stand up and turn his neck round, and to walk and look towards the firelight; all this would hurt him, and he would be too much dazzled to see distinctly those things whose shadows he had seen before. What do you think he would say, if someone told him that what he saw before was foolery, but now he saw more rightly, being a bit nearer reality and turned towards what was a little more real? What if he were shown each of the passing things, and compelled by questions to answer what each one was? Don't you think he would be puzzled, and believe what he saw before was more true than what was shown to him now?"

"Far more," he said.

"Then suppose he were compelled to look towards the real light, it would hurt his eyes, and he would escape by turning them away to the things which he was able to look at, and these he would believe to be clearer than what was being shown to him."

"Just so," said he.

"Suppose, now," said I, "that someone should drag him thence by force, up the rough ascent, the steep way up, and never stop until he could drag him out into the light of the sun, would he not be distressed and furious at being dragged; and when he came into the light, the brilliance would fill his eyes and he would not be able to see even one of the things now called real?"

"That he would not," said he, "all of a sudden."

"He would have to get used to it, surely, I think, if he is to see the things above...."

"... Let him be reminded of his first habitation, and what was wisdom in that place, and of his fellow-prisoners there; don't you think he would bless himself for the change, and pity them?"

"Yes, indeed."...

"Then again," I said, "just consider; if such a one should go down again and sit on his old seat, would he not get his eyes full of darkness coming in suddenly out of the sun?"

"Very much so," said he....

"......And if he should have to compete with those who had been always prisoners, by laying down the law about those shadows while he was blinking before his eyes were settled down - and it would take a good long time to get used to things - wouldn't they all laugh at him and say he had spoiled his eyesight by going up there, and it was not worth-while so much as to try to go up? And would they not kill anyone who tried to release them and take them up, if they could somehow lay hands on him and kill him?"

"That they would!" said he.

"Then we must apply this image, my dear Glaucon," said I, "to all we have been saying. The world of our sight is like the habitation in prison...the ascent and the view of the upper world is the rising of the soul into the world of mind...but God knows if it is really true...." (*The Republic* 514A–517B)

The cave—and the darkened "living-room"—of 2,500 years ago hasn't vanished, though it has been extensively renovated, remodeled, and refurnished. We hold in this book to the ancient Socratic vision of educational enlightenment that once you've stretched a mind even momentarily by liberating it from the cave, it can never completely go back to its old dimensions. In taking ourselves or others out of the cave, we are also on some level taking the cave out of ourselves. In undertaking this educational enlightenment regarding the media environment, we must also maintain a continuous vigilance and awareness of not leaving the cave out into...*another cave*. Many contemporary books on the media are attempts to provide us with a brighter flashlight in the cave. This book hopefully is not one of them.

This book addresses how television effects our bondage to television (Chapter 1); our personhood and our relationship to the world (Chapters 2, 3, and 4); our sense of self and our relationships with others (Chapters 5 and 7); our childhood and parenting (Chapter 6); and our attempts at freedom from this bondage (Chapter 8). Throughout this book, we share how students in our media classes personally encountered these issues in various "experiments" we designed and how they began the journey of awakening to the media matrix, de-hypnotizing themselves and transcending the cave.

Blue vs Red Pill: The Media Matrix

Gurdjieff once said, "If a man wishes to escape from prison the first thing he must do is realize that he is in prison—without that realization, no escape is possible." Everyone in the 1999 film *The Matrix* feels free and feels the familiarity of being themselves as long as they are on-program. In doing the experiments in this book, you will experience the feeling of being "off-program" and hopefully begin to see how already programmed you have been. The moment, the almost-impossible-to-capture moment that you go off-program you personally feel the program inside you.

We address the individuals reading this book as our primary audience because we believe you—like "Neo" in *The Matrix* and "Truman" in *The Truman Show*-- are most acutely in the potential situation and condition of waking up to these damaging forces, these institutions, these administrations, and these self-imprisoning psychologies. We trust both in your *resistance* to seeing and acknowledging these forces—politically in the world and psychologically in yourselves—and in your *basic inquisitiveness*, your openness and will-to-know, your will-to-truth, as it were.

There is a very dramatic scene in the first part of *The Matrix* wherein Morpheus (Lawrence Fishbone) invites Neo (Keneau Reeves) to leave the cave.

MORPHEUS: Do you want to know what it [The Matrix] is Neo? It's the feeling you have had all your life. That feeling that something was wrong with the world. You don't know what it is but it's there, like a splinter in your mind, driving you mad … But what is it? The Matrix is everywhere, it's all around us, here in this room. You can see it out your window, or on your television. You feel it when you go to work, or go to church or pay your taxes. It's the world that has been pulled over your eyes to blind you from the truth.

NEO: What truth?

MORPHEUS: That you are a slave, Neo. That you, like everyone else, was born into bondage … kept inside a prison that you cannot smell, taste, or touch. A prison for your mind. Unfortunately, no one can be told what the Matrix is. You have to see it for yourself.

(http://project.cyberpunk.ru/idb/thematrix_movie_script.html)

We envision our readers like Neo in *The Matrix*, as contemplating the blue or the red pill. Do you want to see or stay comfortably numb? Pick your pill.

1

PARENT TV

Our Third Parent

This book, as we said, is not television. It is a vehicle for an invitation—an invitation to awareness. We will be working to become aware of the nature of our relationship to television and thereby also our relationship to reality, to our society in general, and our self in particular. The current Dalai Lama of Tibet, Tenzin Gyatso, practices meditation four hours a day. The words *media* and *meditation* have a linguistic resonance and kinship. In our experience of the media, we will be exploring how we Americans "do" television watching—how we practice meditation, television meditation—four hours a day. Current A.C. Nielson television statistics for the average American are four hours a day of focused, attentive, exclusive television watching. Combine that together with the TV set also being "on in the background" of the household for another three hours of unfocused, inattentive presence—of a kind of television ambient noise, or second-hand electronic smoke—and we have a total of seven hours a day of direct and diffuse television presence.

This book is a product of our thinking. In the book, we will be *thinking* about television, and we will be *thinking about how we think* about television and how television conditions us to think about ourselves and others. In that sense, this book is "reflective." R. G. Collingwood captures well this concern with being 'reflective' when he talks about his conception of philosophy:

Philosophy is reflective. The philosophizing mind never simply thinks about an object, it always, while thinking about any object, thinks also about its own thought about that object. Philosophy may thus be called thought of the second degree, thought about thought.

(Collingwood 1956:1)

Insofar as we will be thinking about television, we will, of necessity, be thinking about thinking—which is to say we will be displaying a way of thinking and knowing. We will be, by example, modeling a way of *critical* thinking about the media and a way of sociological thinking, or sociologically informed thinking.

Finally, this book on media and television is….*a book*. Regardless of what we say in it—the content—it is an instance, an example, of a certain kind of media. It is an example of the medium of paper-anchored typographic print. It is made up of words on the page. It was composed and *written* by us, and it is being *read* by you. Your *relationship to reading books* will be continuously present, continuously invoked and evoked as you read this work, as will, hopefully, your *relationship to watching television*. We hold, with McLuhan, a synergistic, dynamically interdependent view of the media. "A new medium is never an addition to an old one, nor does it leave the old one in peace" (McLuhan in Benedetti and DeHart 1996:121). The historical emergence of every new media reconfigures all the previously existing media and thereby alters them. It alters their meaning for us, and it alters our experience of them. Television has become deeply revealing of print, books, and reading; that is, a perspicuous investigation of television may "… throw the effects of literacy into sharp and informative relief" (Miller 1971:112).

Because of our media socialization and upbringing, we are already predisposed to seeing television as non-powerful in our lives. This makes the impact of television on us even deeper. Most people believe television is *just* television. This whole book is an argument and an exploration based on the view that television is *not just* television. Rather, television is our third parent. The task really is to have a recognition that television, particularly commercial television, is impactful in ways that ordinarily are never noticed. Guttenberg's printing press invention was impactful in ways that were not recognized for decades and even centuries (McLuhan 1962). In terms of the sociology of knowledge and of epistemology, typographical print became the medium we looked through and that "looking through" is invisible and yet necessary. Even at this very moment, if you the reader somewhat *stop* reading and shift focus onto the p r i n t of these words, they will cease being what they ordinarily are and somewhat become things in and of themselves. We must simultaneously see and transcend looking at the printed word in order to ongoingly accomplish the phenomenon of reading, the *practice* of reading. Note how we visually and mentally transcendently glide smoothly over the surface of the printed letters on the page—noticing them yet not noticing them simultaneously. Reading requires that we actively transcend seeing the literal, graphic ink imprints on the page and yet never disappear them entirely. We must simultaneously notice and transcend the marks into the letters, into the word forms and into the meanings. This is truly an amazing yet ordinary accomplishment/ practice.

> Although the general character of print-intelligence would be known to anyone who would be reading this book, you may arrive at a reasonably detailed definition of it by simply considering what is demanded of you as you read this book. You are required, first of all, to remain more or less immobile for a fairly long time. If you cannot do this (with this or any other book), our culture may label you as anything from hyperkinetic to undisciplined; in any case, as suffering from some sort of intellectual deficiency. The printing press makes rather stringent demands on our bodies as well as our minds. Controlling your body is, however, only a minimal requirement. You must also have learned to pay no attention to the shapes of the letters on the page. You must see through them, so to speak, so that you can go directly to the meanings of the works they form.
>
> (Postman 1985:25)

We are, in this book on television, contending that a similar process happens with regard to watching television.

Our primary intention is for you the *reader* to become *aware* of the *medium* of *television* and alongside that to become aware of the medium of print, to become aware of the *practice* of reading while engaging in reading this book. As Postman put it, "For, like the printing press, television is nothing less than a philosophy of rhetoric. To talk seriously about television, one must therefore talk of epistemology. All other commentary is in itself trivial." (Postman 1985:17). We will be describing a number of experiments in media awareness, epistemological awareness that we have engaged in with our students. We will be inviting you, the reader, to participate in these experiments. In *doing* the experiments or exercises we will be presenting in this book—rather than merely *reading* about them—we hope for you to become aware, or more articulately aware, of the practice of "watching television" while you are "watching television." We also propose asking, "How does the practice of 'watching television' impact our lives when we are not engaged in the practice of 'watching television?'"

The invention and dissemination of our current form of electronic television (and the Internet) has massively altered our relationship to the stable, printed, paper-anchored book. We are beginning to newly recognize that books are "out of print." This change in relationship to print and "print-intelligence" (Postman 1985) has happened globally and in unspecified ways. It is, we hold, a major and peculiar change—a sort of imperceptible yet dislocating experience—perhaps even a traumatizing kind of experience. It's somewhat like the change that occurs if you found out suddenly one day that you are not the biological child of your parents as you had always assumed but that you were in fact adopted. (If you happen to be adopted, just reverse this example.) On one level, everything is exactly as it was before you found this out— your parents are still your parents and you are still you--but on another level, globally, everything changes and begins to reconfigure.

Relationship to TV as Paradigm for Other Life Domains

We want to consider the relationship we have to TV in our contemporary media culture as the paradigm and model for the relationship we have with other domains of our life, that is to say, our relationship with TV models and guides our relationship to other people and to consumer/ material goods. TV impacts our *relationship to relationship*. It channels and funnels our interaction with the world of human relations, with the world of material goods, and with the world of nature. It impregnates our relationship with our self. As we will be arguing throughout this book, we are *deeply* entertained by television; therefore we want to be entertained by our consumer goods and, yes, we even want to be entertained by our human relationships. In *Network* (1976), one of the best films yet made directly about television, the leading character, Diana Christensen (Faye Dunaway), is characterized by her lover, Max Schumacher (William Holden), as "TV incarnate." She habitually and compulsively thinks of all things—her romantic relationship to Max, the social and political events of the day, all her personal and professional experiences—in terms of how they would be as television shows. She very vividly and compulsively transforms everyday reality into dramatic television *on contact*, as King Midas transformed whatever reality he touched into gold. The romantic love relationship between Schumacher (Holden) and Christensen (Dunaway) encapsulates the negative affect television has had on the "television generation." In one scene, Max is asked by his wife whether Diana loves him. He responds, "I'm not sure she is capable of any real feelings. She's television generation. She learned life from Bugs Bunny." Christensen cannot have real intimate, human relationships with other individuals because she has been raised by television, an upbringing dominated by a device that deprives people of grounding in human contact and necessary communication skill development. (more on this in Chapter 5)

One of our undergraduate students caught this acquired television drama skill subtly, almost unconsciously, operating in her own life. (Throughout this book, we will be sharing our students' realizations about our media cave):

Evangeline: I've been thinking about our topic, "Where does the media end and myself begin?" After watching the movie Network I'm not sure. The most eye-opening thing was when the news director, Max Schumacher, was in a relationship with the power hungry lady, Diana Christianson. He realized that she was not capable of seeing life as it is. How she deals with relationships is like a TV show. There is a beginning, commercials in between, and an ending. The ending can be sad or happy, but there always is another show that you can change the channel to see. I think that this is the way a lot of people I know deal with relationships and life in general.

I personally found that it was hard for me to stay in long term relationships without getting bored easily. I felt like there always had to be something happening. Relationships had to be a roller coaster ride in order for me to feel like I had any feelings for the other person. The extreme highs and lows justified that I felt love.... I saw a lot of my past self in the movie. I dealt with relationships the way Diana Christianson dealt with them. She did not understand herself why she was not content with loving someone and being loved.

Our TV training trains us to continuously keep drama *central* and alive in our lives. Our TV training trains us to become more "TV-like."

What does it mean to say, "We become more TV-like?" On one level, we become more like the characters on TV—not the actual working actors; they're working their craft and they're creating, they're *not* watching TV. On another level, we become more like the medium itself of the TV. We become a "TV character," a "TV-person." The way we appear to others imperceptibly changes. We look more like a live TV show, "TV incarnate." The way others appear to us also subtly changes. They seem a bit more like TV characters, or they remind us of TV characters. The world, the environment, looks more and more like the world of TV. So when we turn off the TV and go out, there ceases to be an "out" to go to. When we go out of the cave, we go out *into another cave*. Little by little, indiscernibly, it becomes caves all the way out, and the media matrix becomes real.

Deeply Delusional and In Denial

This book is designed not to show you something new and unknown but rather to engage you in seeing old familiar media in new and unknown ways. Its primary premise is that our acquired relationship to the commercial media is more powerful and more damaging than we have otherwise expected. We want to assert that there is cause for alarm, there is cause for waking up and taking a good, hard look not simply at the media themselves but at our relationship to the media. Somewhat similar to the sustained stance of American culture toward cigarettes for a large stretch of the twentieth century, which was exhaustively analyzed in Brandt's *The Cigarette Century, The Rise, Fall and Deadly Persistence of the Product That Defined America* (Brandt 2007), we contend that as a culture we are in a collective social denial about the depth, dependency, and deception that is at the heart of our relationship to commercial television. We treat *commercial television* as being at the heart of the media culture complex today, the central, solar gravitational point around which all other forms of media revolve, coordinate, and organize themselves. Further, we treat commercial television inside the general theory of socialization. We assert that socialization processes and conditioning processes are centrally at work.

Why is it important to see the self-deception we have been so deeply engaged in regarding our relationship to television and the media in general? Television affects us without our knowing it is affecting us. We hold that *media deception* and *self-deception* are intimately interconnected—more, that there is a deep synergistic relation of inter-destruction incubating and spawning here. Only by cutting through this deep deception can we even begin to access reality, which is to say access the possibility of a life authentically lived. Otherwise we live a life that is not *our* life. We live a mediated, virtual, designer life, mass produced and beamed electronically four hours a day into the command center of our subconscious minds—cloning all of us who are irradiated daily in its all too familiar amniotic glow. As good cave dwellers, we have achieved mastery in the art of ignorance and delusional living.

What is the matter with ignorance and delusional living? Nothing actually, if it is so chosen—as a character in the *Matrxi*, Cypher, ultimately chooses the delusional, virtual reality (Irwin 2002:25). There is a problem (you might call it a political problem) when it is instilled upon the innocent before they can so choose, as seems to be the nature of our television training, especially our childhood television training (more on this in Chapter 6). One relatively small group of people is engaged in instilling this delusional way of being on another relatively large group of people. "Most of television…is as yet controlled by people who are totally controlled by ego, and so the TV's hidden agenda becomes control of you by putting you to sleep, that is to say, making you unconscious" (Tolle 2005:232). TV serves as an institutional vehicle for those who control it to control those who watch it. Eric Fromm, in his criticism of the American TV culture, called this idea "unfreedom" (Fromm 2001). Some of the media power elite, we contend, are cynical about this and to some extent know they are doing it, wherease others are completely taken in by their own delusional being and are transmitting this in good faith. The effects on the receiving end, on us and our children, are still the same.

Denial and Transformation

We hold that discovering how commercialized television—and to some extent "the media"—really works simultaneously and powerfully alters our experience of our self, of how we "work." This method of inquiry and reflection has "denial" and "having a breakthrough regarding denial" built into it—hence the *Platonic Cave* and *The Truman Show* and *Matrix* analogies. Could reality be *that different* from what we have always taken it to be? Could we have personally been in that much delusion regarding reality? Discovering perhaps that we have been in that much delusion regarding ordinary TV reality alters and shifts our view of our self. It alters and shifts our conventional view of our self as having all along been in relation to reality, as someone who has in fact been in a direct, strong, unproblematic relationship with reality.

> There is no more disturbing consequence of the electronic and graphic revolution than this: that the world as given to us through television seems natural, not bizarre. For the loss of the sense of the strange is a sign of adjustment, and the extent to which we have adjusted is a measure of the extent to whish we have been changed. Our culture's adjustment to the epistemology of television is by now all but complete.
>
> (Postman 1985:80)

The thrust of what we would like our readers to come away with is a more critically vigilant awareness and stance toward the impact of the commercial media. Vigilance as an investigative quality and mode of research is highly alert, attentive, and rigorously, globally suspicious. Where most of us practice gullibility toward the media—they just are, they are our friends, they are transparently neutral, they affect others but not me—vigilance pushes us to be ever suspicious, ever distrusting, ever on guard.

Why? Why cultivate a vigilant attitude? Why practice a kind of *methodological paranoia*? Because a neutral, information driven inquiry will not have the force, the emotional momentum, to cut through the deeply layered conditioning that our media culture has woven into our collective psyches since childhood. Vigilance is somehow necessary to cut through the deeply weighted resistance toward disequilibrium, toward the spiraling into a deeply disturbing unfamiliarity that we as culturally conditioned beings have been trained to avoid at all costs.

Recall Socrates in Plato's "Parable of the Cave": "Suppose…that someone should drag him thence by force, up the rough ascent, the steep way up … would he not be distressed and furious at being dragged…" (*Republic* 517B). Only the most emotionally charged psychic-dissolving solvent could hope to penetrate our resistance to anything threatening our familiar cave environment.

When we reinvestigate and reframe our relationship with the electronic media, primarily with commercial TV, both as we were growing up and now, we may make a discovery of a similar order of magnitude: *We may discover that TV has been our parent*, that we have been deeply formed and shaped by this bonding relationship to TV. Parenting has changed drastically with the introduction of television. Prior to the introduction of TV into the modern domestic family household, "parents" and "parenting" were significantly different enterprises from what they are today. Growing up in a television household, our parents aren't the same parents they would be without television present. To exaggerate the point, *our parents aren't our parents; the TV is our parent* or, more accurately, *TV is our third parent* (McKibben 1992). Somewhat "Stepford wife-ish," we may discover that we have been to a great degree raised by a virtual machine, an animated robot. We now have real relationships with unreal characters and a personal relationship with an impersonal technology.

Television and the Theology of Parenting

Behind and alongside our experience of the parent-person, we discover that there is *a machine*. In this book, we argue that *the blending of TV and the parent category is deep and powerful.* In terms of the sociology and psychology of religion—Freud's seminal works here are *Totem and Taboo* (1918), *Moses and Monotheism* (1939), and *The Future of an Illusion* (1928)—we can see that for many adherents of the world's religions, the concept of *God* is, at bottom, *parental:* "…the real relationship of God and man is that of parent and child" (Fox 1934:133). The parental relationship, the parental figure, is—from the infant and child's perspective—the most powerful and meaningful, the most influential relationship on the planet. Whoever or whatever can influence this relationship, whoever or whatever can infiltrate and affect this primal, parental relationship can deeply impact the world, can, to some degree, define the world. TV does that. Television technology and the family and social relations it anchors have had and continue to have an almost totemic power over its children. (More on this in Chapter 6.) It is experienced as an ordinary yet unnoticed, almost molecular, splicing of the personal and the machine. In terms of the primitive psychology of our childhood, if the parent says it, it is so (or, in the mode of childhood resistance, it is *not* so.). If the TV shows it, it is so (there is almost *no* mode of resistance for the child toward the TV).

Television is *a personal, intimate machine* and, at the same time, it *is also a parent machine.* The feeling tone of the pair-bond that gets set up with the television has more in common with parental bonding than with sibling pair bonding. The awe-filled, phenomenal cult of celebrity in the United States and probably worldwide is fueled by this same complex reservoir of relationship energy (i.e., how we relate to our parents, and more, how we relate to God). We contend that the parental relation, the god–higher power relation, is operative here.

Denying Parenting and TV Influence

We resist taking seriously the effects that television has on us. That resistance is a central topic of concern in this book. It is our contention that resistance to taking seriously the effects of television on our development and our overall relationship with reality is the hallmark of our media programming. Our media programs us to resist taking seriously its impact on us. Our media experience is such that it eliminates its effect upon us *after* having that effect. It has a certain magical disappearing dimension to it. "It's just television." "It's just entertainment." "It's just advertising." We are contending that that view is the equivalent of saying that our parents, our upbringing and socialization, don't really affect us all that much. Of course, we also resist taking seriously the effects that our parents have had on us. Part of their impact is to leave us in a state of denial toward the enormity of that impact. From a cynical, political perspective, if I can program you in such a way as to convince you that you're doing what you are doing solely or even primarily because you are freely and spontaneously doing it and *not* because I have programmed you to do it, then my programming is powerful indeed.

Our relationship with our parents had an enormous influence on our formation. It colors all aspects of our life and even how we think about our parents and about parenting. Our interactional patterns get formed through our interaction with our parents. We are imprinted by our parents as models for how to be, how to act and behave and interact. They are always broadcasting to us, their children, ways of being. Whatever else they are busy doing, they are always also modeling ways of being in the world, ways of responding to situations. Television is always also modeling ways of being in the world. It models this through the content we see on the screen directly but, more powerfully, it models its technological nature— it's capacity to display images and captivate those who encounter it. With our human parents, we have a back-and-forth interactional field always happening. With our TV parent, we have a numb, absorbing relationship. Our TV parent is always there....there to entertain us.

What We Would Like Readers of This Book to Realize

In brief, these are the main realizations that we hope to provoke in our readers:

- We have been influenced and programmed by the media and-we-don't-believe-we-have.
- The programming we have internalized from the media is not for the enhancement of our life and happiness but rather for the commercial benefit of the established ruling orders. (The established ruling groups are themselves caught up in and under the spell of the media dreamscape they labor to help sustain into continued existence.)
- The purpose of this programming is to reinforce into continued existence the status quo and to deepen and expand it.
- The more we watch, the less we know. Or, more precisely, the more we watch, the less we know while simultaneously thinking we know more.
- Our conceptions and expectations of relationships, love, and beauty have been altered deeply by commercial media.
- The more we fill our self and our life with media, the less we actually live our own life.
- Within our media culture, media takes priority over experience, over direct personal or collective experience. Our experience of media is

that media takes priority over experience. In the back of our media-matrixed minds, if you watch it, you have experienced/done it.

- We can transform our relationship to the media.
- We can ourselves produce media in such a way that it wakes people up rather than puts them more deeply asleep.
- What is to be done? Live differently. Wake up.

The Media Monopoly and the Monopoly of Media

Why should we want to undertake this kind of inquiry? What is the purpose of becoming sociologically and psychologically aware of the media? What is the purpose of becoming aware of the power and the influence of the media on our experience of reality and on our experience of identity? The way we experience reality *is our* identity. It is better to be aware than not to be aware. It is also better to be aware of the nature of awareness. Again, why? It gives us freedom. What type of freedom? The freedom to *be* free; not to *have* freedom—like another commodity we buy—but to *be* free, to access the being of freedom. Why is this so necessary today in the field of televisual culture? Media frame the outlook of the world we live in. Through it, we are imprinted into the framework of our reality. What we know about what is happening in the world, how the weather will be, who our enemies or friends are, what we should buy and wear are just a few of the ways the media helps shape our reality. Media critics even tell us what to think of a TV show, movie, or piece of art. Unfortunately, these messages are not all done explicitly; most of media's influence comes at us in hidden packages. The all-encompassing saturation of media in our society, what Bagdikian has called *The Media Monopoly*, is reminiscent of the unitary power of the Medieval church. In the Medieval Age, the Christian church was the all-pervasive, ruling environment. In our Media Age, that institution and belief structure is commercial television. In our historical age, it is commercial television that both supports and degrades and also threatens the reality structure of human life on our planet. It is commercial television that captivates, imprints, imprisons, and programs our contemporary psychology.

Peter Weir's 1998 satirical movie, *The Truman Show*, starring Jim Carrey opened around the country. This movie was a powerful example of the influence the media matrix we live in has on our lives. In the movie, the main character, Truman (True-man), the first human being ever to be owned by a corporation, born in front of a live television audience, lives a manufactured, mediated life or, rather, lives a real life in a massive, manufactured media reality, namely the world's largest television set—the size of a small nation (or large cave). His parents, wife, friends, associates are all, unbeknownst to him, paid professional actors performing roles in a "reality" television show. Truman is the only person who does not know his life, his performance, is not real but contrived, scripted, controlled, and manipulated for dramatic and commercial purposes. The director, Christof (Ed Harris)—the creative, conspiratorial, paternalistic mastermind behind the show—controls what happens to Truman. On this enormous manufactured television set, Truman's life was everyone else's job and, in terms of "Reality TV," Truman's life was the world's entertainment. His cave-life was fabricated and planned by someone else. Truman's life is a provocative analogy of all of our lives in the Media Age. To what extent is someone controlling what we think and do? Are the network programmers, news producers, and advertising executives somehow controlling how we think and act as an individual and as a society? To what extent is our life manufactured, like Truman's? Truman eventually recognized what was happening in his life. He woke up and fought against the web of illusions. He rebelled. He left the cave. As individuals in a media-saturated society walking our pathways through the immense environmental density of television, we too can become aware of the extent of the media's role in our life. After examining media's influence on our own experience of life, we feel each individual must, like Truman, choose what to do.

TV as Institution Versus TV as Practice

In our conventional view of society, we believe social *institutions* "are," they just simply exist; whereas *practices* are what we "do." A practice is in some sense a voluntary action and also an accomplishment. It is repeated again and again. Rather then holding that an institution just is, that it somehow just exists, we want to ask, "How do we *practice* institutions?" This question in turn leads to "How do we practice culture?" "How do we practice society?" We also want to include in this investigation "How do we practice our identity?" "How do we practice our identity as a cultural, social institution?" or, perhaps, "How is my 'I' a social institution?"

In this inquiry, we want to become aware of the *practice* of television; primarily the practice of television and secondarily the practice of media in general. *To become aware of the practice of television is simultaneously to become aware of television as a practice.* So we are engaged specifically in seeing television as a practice and, in general, seeing media as a practice. Why? What is the good of seeing television as a practice? This approach will help us to experience our active participation in the institution of television and see how we, as it were, "co-create" television. Inside our media cave, we might come to see that it is also we who are stoking the fire and carrying along the items above the puppet wall that are throwing the shadows on the cave wall.

What is the good of this practice of becoming aware of practices? It pushes our growth and development. It furthers the truth. What's the good of furthering the truth? What type of truth? What's the truth of this truth? As we mentioned somewhat like cigarette smokers in the 1950s, the truth of the situation is we are in a profound confusion about the truth of television. We are in a profound confusion about the truth of television and the media and in a profound confusion about the truth of confusion. This book is a small exercise in de-confusing our relationship to the practice of television and the practice of media. To go from unconsciously accomplishing a practice to an awareness of unconsciously accomplishing a practice is, we believe, a step toward moving from imprisonment to freedom.

When we are *in* confusion, we are not in clear awareness. We are dulled over, benumbed. We are bewitched and cross eyed. We are in distraction. Television allows us to be in a state of distraction while experiencing it as entertainment and information. It is a soothing, opiated distraction, a form of being intoxicated on distraction and distractedness. As a daily practice (four hours a day), television helps us to cultivate a distracted state of mind so that we don't directly and clearly relate to reality. "A short attention span makes all your perceptions and relationships shallow and unsatisfying. Whatever you do, whatever action you perform in that state, lacks quality, because quality requires attention" (Tolle 2005:232).

A Safe Experience of Danger

The renowned Vietnamese spiritual teacher and meditation master, Thich Nhat Hahn, has commented pointedly on our familiar, ordinary TV crisis:

> Do you ever find yourself watching an awful TV program, unable to turn it off? The raucous noises, explosions of gunfire, are upsetting. Yet you don't get up and turn it off. Why do you torture yourself in this way? Don't you want to close your windows? Are you frightened of solitude—the emptiness and the loneliness you may find when you face yourself alone?
>
> Watching a bad TV program, we *become* the TV program. We are what we feel and perceive. If we are angry, we are the anger. If we are in love, we are love. If we look at a snow-covered mountain peak, we are the mountain. We can be anything we want, so why do we open our windows to bad TV programs made by sensationalist producers in search of easy money, programs that make our hearts pound, our fists tighten, and leave us exhausted? Who allows such TV programs to be made and seen even by the very young? We do! We are too undemanding, too ready to watch whatever is on the screen, too lonely, lazy, or bored to create our own lives. We turn on the TV and leave it on, allowing someone else to guide us, shape us, and destroy us. Leaving ourselves in this way is leaving our fate in the hands of others who may not be acting responsibly .
>
> (Nhat Hahn. *Peace is Every Step*: 13)

The Diagnostic and Statistical Manual for Mental Disorders (DSM-IV) is the authoritative text/manual used by therapists to formally diagnose clients with reference to mental disorders. The first criterion that is used to determine the presence and diagnosis of "Post Traumatic Stress Disorder" in the DSM-IV is,

> A. The person has been exposed to a traumatic event in which both of the following were present: (1) the person experienced, witnessed, or was confronted with an event or events that involved actual or threatened death or serious injury, or a threat to the physical integrity of self or others (2) the person's response involved intense fear, helplessness, or horror.
>
> (DSM-IV-TR 2000:467)

In reference to television, we are in some sense *trained to see it as harmless*, as ordinary, as mundane. Our actual experience of it, however, is not ordinary, harmless, and mundane. It is somehow a continuous visual alarm. As the car alarm or the fire alarm catches and captivates our ears and our consciousness, so the TV catches and captivates our consciousness. "*Why is it so hard to stop watching?*" It is easier never to have turned the television on than, once on, to turn it off. It compels continued use. What compels our attention, above all else, is danger and alarm.

TV is visual danger, without itself being dangerous; it is *a safe experience of danger.* After all, we watch TV in the safety of our own home. We don't want to have a dangerous experience of danger. We want a pretend experience of danger. With media, we bathe ourselves in images of life and death or, rather, entertainment fantasy images of life and death—and we come away cleansed. Watching others die does one good. Watching others get "blown away" does one good. What sort of good is this? What sort of death is this that we watch? It is not real, therefore it is okay. It is not real, it is pretend, therefore it is appealing, fun, stimulating. On some level, it teaches that death and mortality are not real.

A good portion of television is run by the imagineers of disaster and danger. Excitement, danger, thrills, suspense—all done for the pursuit of attention: the capturing and holding of attention. Why? What is the good of it? To capture attention is to capture value. Or, rather, that which is successful in capturing attention is defined as valuable. Why would you want to capture attention? Capturing attention is the necessary foundation for all communication, for without attention, there is no communication. (Attention makes communication possible.) However, because danger and death make for more attention-captivating TV, thinking and normal human relationships are almost banished from the media. These do not create attention.

This is the situation of watching "über alles." It s a certain kind of watching, a watching that is highly safe. It is safe in the home. It does not have the ever-present subtle threat of the public space, the public arena. All the windows and doors are secured. Perhaps the phone is turned off. *To watch is a form of safety. To watch danger inside this form of safety is somehow doubly safe.* We are in a form of safety and exposing ourselves to danger at the same time. We are watching people in all kinds of dangerous and violent situations. We are watching all kinds of drama. We watch their life *to forget our life*. We watch the drama in their life to momentarily forget the anxieties of our own life. The drama in their life pulls us out of our preoccupation with our own life's worries and concerns. If we are personally engaged in the middle of an emotional drama or in the middle of some real danger, the last thing we can do is "watch TV."

Critique Versus Media Therapy: How is the Media My Problem?

What is the most effective attitude to take in regard to an inquiry into the media? On the one hand, we have the wildly critical, paranoid approach that operates in a vacuum: This is wrong, bad, and harmful and ought to be immediately changed. This disconnected form of critique in not grounded in the actual and ongoing accomplishment of the media. On the other hand, we don't want to merely become spokesmen for the already existing: What is, is justified *because* it is. If we are completely embedded in the already existing and the already achieved, it is beyond critique and beyond reflection.

Critical reflection acknowledges the existing state of affairs while simultaneously leaving room to see its contingency: to acknowledge its existence and to acknowledge its managed precariousness at the same time. It is, but it need not be the way it is: It is one possible arrangement, one possible manifestation among many others.

How does critique of the media relate to therapy, to what we might call *media therapy*? How is it different from a traditional political assault on the media? How is media therapy the middle way between mere criticism and passive acceptance? For therapy to be effective, it must begin with discontent over the existing situation. Without discontent or, rather, without the conscious awareness of discontent, the project of therapy and the practice of therapy would not be undertaken. In terms of our contemporary media dynamics, we hold that both *discontent* and *denial* play a major role. How so denial? If we are merely discontent, we need primarily to "adjust" our self to the situation or adjust the situation to our self, or achieve some form of "compromise." If we are in denial, then what is most needed is an *awareness of* our denial.

We need awareness that we are *in* denial, which is to say we need to become aware that we have been invested in *not seeing*, in deceiving ourselves. The self-deception of denial, the using of the energy and skill of denial to deny denial is at the threshold of *therapy for addiction*—therapy for the phenomenon of addiction. Whereas the purpose of therapy is to accomplish some form of clarity and freedom, the purpose of commercial, advertising media is to instill some form of confusion and attachment.

In the next chapter, we look at why in the world of television no one ever really watches television or why there is no cave inside the cave.

2

IDENTITY TV

You Are What You Watch

The eminent French sociologist, Piere Bourdieu, once said while being interviewed on television, "I'd like to try and pose here, on television, a certain number of questions about television. This is a bit paradoxical since, in general, I think that you can't say much on television, particularly not about television" (Bourdieu 1998:13).

Have you ever noticed *that nobody on TV ever watches TV?* A short glance or two perhaps but no real, sustained, trance-eyed watching, hours on end, the way we, the television audience, are watching. We watch television to see what life is like for people who don't watch television. As we mentioned, surveys tell us that most Americans have their TV sets on in the background an average of seven hours a day (Gitlin 2002:15–17). In his 1978 work on television, *Four Arguments for the Elimination of Television*, the renegade advertising executive, Jerry Mander, reported that

> According to the A.C. Nielson Company, 95 percent of the U.S. population watches some TV everyday. No day goes by without a "hit" of television, which indicates the level of engagement, or addiction, that people feel for the medium.
>
> Nielson reports that the average American home has a television on for nearly eight hours per day. The average American adult watches TV nearly five hours per day... But if the *average* person is watching five hours per day, then roughly half of the U.S. population is watching *more* than five hours.
>
> (Mander 1978:76)

As Mander reported in 1978, so Professor Todd Gitlin reported in 2002:

> Overall … 'watching TV' is the dominant leisure activity of Americans, consuming 40 percent of the average person's free time as a primary activity [when people give television their undivided attention]. Television takes up more than half of our free time if you count … watching TV while doing something else like eating or reading … [or] when you have the set on but you aren't paying attention to it. Sex, race, income, age and marital status make surprisingly little difference in time spent. Neither, at this writing, has the Internet diminished total media use, even if you don't count the Web as part of the media. While Internet users do watch 28 percent less television, they spend more time than nonusers playing video games …
>
> (Gitlin 2002:16)

Children spend as much time in front of the set as at school. So here is, by far, the biggest leisure-time pursuit of Americans, yet *inside the television world it doesn't exist*. Inside the cave there is no cave. The world we watch when we watch TV does not reflect the world we live in as we watch TV. When you think about it, this is hardly surprising. What could be more boring than watching somebody on TV watching TV?

In terms of the "reality TV" shows of recent years, *Big Brother* unconsciously addressed this theme in the very heart of its structure.

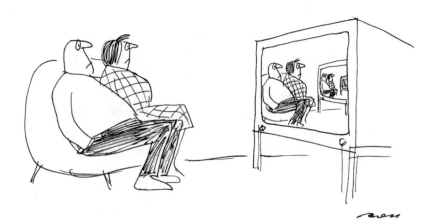

Within the *Big Brother* house, contact with the outside world was limited; there were no phones, televisions, radios, or computers in the house, which the web page described as a "back-to-basics" environment... Indeed, the paradoxical absence of the mass media (in a show created by and for these media) was described as a return not only to face-to-face community but as an incitation to participatory forms of entertainment. The house guests, as the show's host, Julie Chen, observed in the premier episode, had to find ways of entertaining themselves rather than relying on the products of the entertainment industry...The *Big Brother* house thus *became a mass media experiment in watching people deprived of the mass media.*

(Andrejevic 2004:118; emphasis mine)

In the background of our habitual four hours a day of focused television watching, there lies, as we mentioned here, an unsettling paradox: We watch television to see what life is like for people who don't watch television. This is a practice that is truly non-reflexive, that is truly incapable of doing what it is doing and being aware of what it is doing simultaneously. The primary function of the "reality TV" show is drama with a strong voyeuristic personal element that has made it flourish. We watch TV to "relax," as we say. The people in the shows that we are watching are not themselves "relaxing." As a nation, collectively we watch TV four hours a day, yet the people in "TV nation" aren't watching TV.

What we really wish to emphasize here is the phenomenal denial mode that we must activate to individually practice and socially participate in this TV culture. The latent function of commercial, mass television, entertainment media is to somehow hide itself from us as a distinctive institutional form. It must appear natural and, in a sense, invisible. What the commercial mass media must at all times keep concealed is their artificial nature. They are an accomplished artifice and an accomplished cultural practice in a similar way that—to pick a dramatically negative analogy—smoking cigarettes was/is an artificial, accomplished cultural practice. The corporate-sponsored media enterprise enlists our participation in this television-watching practice. Television watching is both participating and consuming. The best possible ideal type of viewer are those who never bring their participation in this practice into their conscious awareness. In terms of our cigarette-smoking analogy, for a large part of the twentieth century, while the culture as a whole was inside the denial mode, smoking appeared as "normal," "harmless," "ordinary," as "ok," "cool." "Nearly half of all adults were smokers in the years before 1970" (Brandt 2007:5). It took a lot of collective social action to begin to come out of this corporate-sponsored denial trance and see this cultural practice as artificial—and not only artificial but as toxic and deadly.

Big Brother says let's watch people "deprived" of television and "deprived" of mass media. A little later in this chapter, we describe the "Un-TV" experiment in media awareness that we assigned our students. In the "Un-TV" experiment, we will talk about how we did something similar yet fundamentally different with our students. We asked students to *not* watch TV for a designated period of time and become aware of what they were doing; that is to say, we assigned them to consciously watch TV for 15 minutes *without turning it on* and to investigate and become aware of what they actually experienced. With *Big Brother* we, as the TV-viewing audience, were invited to watch people deprived of television, but all this, of course, was actually *just more television*. This doesn't invite reflexive awareness of the actual cultural practice of watching television. If you "deprive" people of watching television and then watch them on television to see how they do with this deprivation, you are never really consciously *questioning* television: You are just *extending* unconscious television watching. Rather than leaving the cave, you are watching a shadow of yourself leaving the cave.

This unnoticed dimension of the practice of television watching was pointedly addressed in Barbara Ehrenreich's *The Worst Years of Our Lives.*

> So why do we keep on watching? The answer, by now, should be perfectly obvious: we love television *because television brings us a world in which television does not exist.* In fact, deep in their hearts, this is what the spuds crave most: a rich, new, participatory life, in which people walk outside and banter with the neighbors, where there is adventure, possibility, danger, feeling, all in natural color, stereophonic sound, and three dimensions, without commercial interruptions, and starring... us.
>
> (Ehrenreich 1990:17; emphasis added)

Cinematic films—movies—we think, are not quite this way. They often reflect back upon themselves. Scores of films have been made about making films. There have even been films in which the characters come off the screen and start to participate in real life. In a movie, it isn't unusual to have movie characters shown at the movies, with shots alternating between the screen and the audience. This difference is puzzling. Perhaps it is because movies are an occasional thrill in our lives whereas television is a daily drug, infinitely less interesting or original. Movies invite us to dream, television invites us into a state of somnambulance.

> TV is a pipeline to the modern world...that does not mean that TV merely reflects our society. By virtue of its omnipotence, it also constantly reinforces certain ideas. *It is less an art form than the outlet for a utility*— like the faucet on a sink that connects you to the river, the TV links you to a ceaselessly flowing stream of information, and that very ceaselessness makes it different from a play or a movie.
>
> (McKibben 1992:17; emphasis added)

The fact that TV characters never watch TV is part of *television's systematic, institutional, and total denial of the influence of TV in American life*. Whenever we look to television to enlighten us on this subject, it sidesteps instantly away.

As soon as you look critically *at* television, it changes your experience *of* television. The purpose of our reflections in this book is *to call your critical attention to the power of television, and indeed, of all the commercial mass media, on your life*. We do this under the banner once succinctly stated by the late sociologist, Herbert Marcuse, "Consciousness of oppression is the precondition of all liberation."

Most of us frequently fall back on television to dull our feelings of self-doubt, to give us escape from a life that is too rushed and pressured: "the trance we turn on television to create" (McKibben 1992:199). However, we are caught in a vicious circle here because many of our self-doubts stem directly from media culture—the very culture to which we turn for escape. The contemporary novelist, David Foster Wallace, captured this in his essay on television:

> The appeal of watching television has always involved fantasy. And contemporary TV has gotten vastly better at enabling the viewer's fantasy that he can transcend the limitations of individual human experience, that he can be inside the set ...

Of course, the downside of TV's big fantasy is that it's just a fantasy. As a Treat, my escape from the limits of genuine experience is neato. As a steady diet, though, it can't help but render my own reality less attractive … render me less fit to make the most of it (because I spend all my time pretending I'm not in it), and render me ever more dependent on the device that affords escape from just what my escapism makes unpleasant.

(Wallace 1997:75).

As for our highly stressed and pressured lifestyle, it too stems in large part from media values and media's view of reality. "Ours is the first society in history of which it can be said that life has moved *inside* media. The average person, watching television for five hours per day, is physically engaged with—looking at and experiencing— a *machine*" (Mander 1991:76) and "…The media flow into the home—not to mention outside—has swelled into a torrent of immense force and constancy, an accompaniment *to* life that has become a central experience *of* life" (Gitlin 2002:17).

Media mediate not only between a reality beyond our immediate experience and ourselves; they mediate between us and our self-images, affecting our most intimate experience of our self. Media also don't just report and respond to our culture and society; they are a major player in shaping that which they pretend only to report on. In this inquiry, we want to concentrate not only on what media tell us but on what media hide from us. As Michael Parenti has said, "The entertainment media are the make-believe media; they make us believe" (Parenti 1992:1). The media have become the medium of explanation for our reality. Our interpreting consciousness is channeled through media reference points and, as Postman argues, our televisual electronic media has now become our epistemology (Postman 1985).

Un-TV: You Are What You Watch—The Exercise

David: I have been watching TV for 18 years, and I had to not-watch it for 15 minutes to realize what it is I've been doing.

Erika: If the TV is on, I can watch it for hours. When it is off, I can't stand watching it.

"How many of you know how to watch television?" we asked our college class one day. After many bewildered and silent moments, cautiously, suspiciously, one by one, everyone hesitantly raised their hands.

Such questions seriously listened to tend to momentarily short-circuit our conventional consensus trance and provoke us at least into beginning to question ordinary social life and social practices from a more sociological and ethnomethodological perspective. Such questions can generate a mild, momentary experience of "mind-stop" and "de-socialization." In a sense, it's not the answers that are important but rather gaining access to a way of questioning, a way of seeing, and a way of "waking up" as the Buddhists might say.

Regarding the question to our classes about "knowing how to watch TV," we soon acknowledged that we were all "experts," as Garfinkel (1967) would say, in the practice and accomplishment of watching television. In our ordinary experience, we watch television. The purpose of our Un-TV experiment was to provoke us into *seeing* television, to "see," rather than to merely "watch."

The exercise we devised to explore and reveal the individual practice and societal culture of "watching television" had a number of different dimensions.

1. Count the technical events during a 10-minute span of any show you chose.
2. In this particular experimental odyssey, we are going to be exploring how we subject ourselves on a daily basis to the overwhelming sirens' song of TV entertainment, the great electronic siren, and so, like Homer's Odysseus, we will need to strap ourselves to the ship's mast—the mast being, in this case, counting technical events. For 10 minutes, simply count the technical events that occur while you are watching any show. This is a TET, or technical events test, as Mander discusses it in *Four Arguments for the Elimination of Television* (1978:303–312). What is a technical event? We've all seen TV cameras in banks, jewelry, and liquor stores, and the like that simply record what's in front of them. This is what we will call "pure TV." It's interesting for a moment but soon becomes quite boring. Anything other than pure TV is a technical event. The camera

zooms up; that's a technical event. You're watching someone talking and suddenly you are switched to another person responding; that's a technical event. A car is moving down the road, and you also hear music playing; that's a technical event. Simply count the number of times you see or hear a cut, zoom, superimposition, voiceover, words on the screen, fade in/out, and so on. Try to include at least one commercial break within your 10 minutes.

3. Watch any TV show of your choice for 10 minutes without turning the sound on.

4. Watch any news program for 10 minutes without turning the sound on.

5. Rather than watching TV, watch someone watching TV for 10 minutes. It is best if they don't know their being watched. At the end of that 10 minutes, try to neutrally and simply, yet abruptly, switch off the TV set and observe what happens.

6. Finally, watch television for 15 minutes *without turning it on.*

With this exercise, the time requirements are extremely important. This experiment is to be done with "Beginner's Mind," a term taken from the Japanese Zen master Shunryu Suzuki, Roshi (Suzuki 1970). Beginner's mind is a fresh, hollow, open, flexible mind that doesn't know in advance what it is going to experience. It is, in essence, the opposite of "expert's mind," which is so pre-filled with knowledge, opinions, views, and sophistication that it can't see anything new and fresh. Beginner's mind is very childlike in its open alertness to what is going on. The final instructions are, while doing these experimental exercises, "Don't daydream, fantasize, or drift off. Don't remember your past nor plan your future. Stay present. Stay in the now. Observe what goes on within you and without you. See what you can see." (You can perhaps see the analogies to meditation instruction here.) At this point, we would urge readers to undertake the experiment personally on their own (which, of course, requires you to stop and interrupt your reading).

Anger and Resistance: "What's the Purpose of This!?"

Author McGrane vividly remembers once, after giving his students these instructions for their television experiment, one exceedingly irate student practically shouted out to him, "What's the purpose of this!?" Before he could respond, another student replied to her with the equally charged question, "What's the purpose of asking for a purpose? With these exercises maybe we're beginning to go beyond the fixed idea that everything has to have a purpose." As instructors, both of us have experienced a good deal of anger and resistance from students in our media classes. Trying to break out of the cave-matrix is not easy, and resistance to going off-program is strong.

The foregoing students' observations were very prescient. In studying aspects of media and society and by engaging in exercises in de-socialization, we were beginning to cut through our compulsive need to have a purpose. Somewhat like the Zen novice practicing zazen meditation, the students began to understand—slightly anyway—this *need* to understand, this somewhat compulsive *need* to have a purpose. They also saw that when they let go of this habitual security, when they actually experienced for a short time that their activity had no prescribed purpose, when they accessed more directly beginner's mind, their awareness and sensitivity, insight, and intelligence became acute in a way they had never experienced before. They were beginning to cut through the socialization process and opened up more to becoming de-hypnotized.

In examining the results of this exercise, one of the first things that arises consistently is, as we said, the students' anger and resentment at being made to do such a thing. Their anger and resentment have a very different quality from that which can arise, say, in response to the quantity of reading or homework assignments or the writing requirements. Palmer, in his work, *The Courage to Teach*, says,

> Good education may leave students deeply dissatisfied, at least for a while. I do not mean the dissatisfaction that comes from teachers who are inaudible, incoherent, or incompetent. But students who have been well served by good teachers may walk away angry—angry that their prejudices have been challenged and their sense of self shaken. That sort of dissatisfaction may be a sign that real education has happened...It can take years for a student to feel grateful to a teacher who introduces a dissatisfying truth.
>
> (Palmer 1998:94)

Their distinctive anger and resistance, we think, are quite good and useful—insofar as students notice it and then inquire into and examine the sources causing it. In studying media and society, we often unconsciously assume we are studying "them"—but we are not. We are studying ourselves and, though we may not resist that *abstract idea*, we dislike that *personal experience*. Doing sociology, from this point of view, makes us uncomfortable and angry. We start examining the illusions we live by in contrast to the realities we live in, and we can often come uncomfortably close to that uncanny, slightly paranoid and hunted feeling so well expressed by the Russian existentialist philosopher, Shestov: "It is not man who pursues truth, but truth man."

One frequent expression of this anger is the statement "I wasted fifteen minutes of my time!" Is it possible that wasting time is very valuable in examining the time-pressure imperatives of our socialization process? After some discussion, all of the students invariably admit to having wasted a lot more than 15 minutes in front of the TV set. What is going on, really, with this anger about watching TV without turning it on? Some of the initial responses are revealing:

Kevin: I was sitting there. I was getting angry. I was doing nothing. It was about this time that I realized that whenever I watched TV with it on I was still essentially doing nothing. The difference was that when the TV was on I had something to concentrate on. TV seems to give a guilt-free way of doing nothing.

Adam: I was not being entertained therefore I was angry. I wasn't bored because I wasn't doing anything, rather I was bored because TV wasn't doing anything for me. It wasn't entertaining me. I found it very frustrating not being able to have my TV set communicate with me, and then it dawned on me that the reason I was feeling frustrated was because we have become conditioned to think that the TV is our best friend.

Lisa: In the next fifteen minutes, I stared at the television after turning it off. The first thing I saw was my own reflection; and something horribly shocking occurred to me: how much of what I see in myself is real? How much of me has been shaped or altered by watching TV all these years? I then realized how much I really needed to unlearn before I can see myself in the light I was intended to be seen.

In our Un-TV experiment, we engaged in "stopping the world" by "stopping the television" (Castaneda 1972:ix). As a society, we view television as real. We watch our wars and our "smart bombs" on the same TV sets as our football games. The American sociologist W. I. Thomas taught us long ago, "If humans define situations as real, they become real in their consequences." From an ethnomethodological perspective, in our Un-TV experiment, we bracketed the natural attitude of realism while watching TV (Heritage 1984:38–43). That is, we attempted to see how the practice-and-institution called "watching TV" is a contingent, highly active, precarious, yet routinized, ongoing accomplishment rather than a passive, inert, and transparent perception of an external object.

One student put it rather succinctly regarding the experience of watching the TV for 15 minutes while it was not turned on: "If the TV is on I can watch it for hours. When it is off I can't stand watching it." Our question is, "What is going on here?" What transformation occurs to our sense of time and space? A good part of our life is spent sitting inside our television experience (four hours a day). By unifying human beings within its framework and by centralizing experience within itself, TV virtually *replaces* environment (Mander 1977). It accelerates our alienation from nature, thereby inducing the destruction of nature.

With this exercise with television, we are at the threshold of the possibility of stepping outside of the Platonic Cave. We are dealing here with the social construction of reality (Berger and Luckman 1966) and, if this unnoticed work of accomplishing and constructing ordinary social life is experienced personally regarding the practice of watching commercial TV, it can be extended with great liberating force and effectiveness to other media practices and to other social practices and other social institutions, for example, the school or the economy.

Craig: Critical television viewing is unkind to TV. Approaching the experience as an exercise in empiricism, that is, not turning off the brain at the same moment the screen lights up, the absurdity of the medium is glaringly apparent. Taken purely as an artifact, the descriptive phrase "haunted box" fits and fits well. Watching with a beginner's mindset is, all in all, a nauseating process. When the audio masking is stripped away, an interesting difference between shows and commercials becomes immediately apparent. The commercials have much higher production values and input than the programs they sponsor. Their film-like quality is a huge contrast to the shot-on-video quality of many current network sitcoms. The characterizations of the inhabitants of the commercials are much more animated and vital than the wooden portrayals of the poor souls stranded in the substandard world for the ten minutes in between the ads. The ad-people may have waxy buildup on their floors and odiferous body parts but they do have the newest and improvedest of everything and anything and everything is color coordinated right down to the curtains and the baby. The commercial announcements appear more REAL than the fare they divide.

For this exercise, students were asked to actually watch TV, to consciously watch TV. Insofar as this is sort of "Zen and the art of TV watching," we said to them, "We want you to watch TV with acute awareness, mindfulness and precision, seeing what you watch, watching what you see. Examine 'the trance we turn on television to create' (McKibben 1992:199). Usually we don't watch the TV itself, just the screen or, rather, just what's on the screen. So for this experiment, we want you to watch TV, not a show or a program, just TV. This experiment is about *observing* television, scientifically, with beginner's mind, rather than "watching television" passively, with expert's programmed mind. Consider that, when you are driving down the highway, you can't really closely observe your windshield. That is way too dangerous. You have to look *through* the windshield to the road. Ordinarily, if you are watching TV, you can't also observe and experience the experience of watching TV. When we watch TV, we rarely pay attention to the details of the event; in fact, we rarely pay attention. This experiment is designed to make "watching TV" *into* an experience, an experience we can notice, rather than an unconsciousness, an absence of experience—which for most of us most of the time it mostly is.

Sue: Everyday when I come home from school, I race to the television set to watch my favorite noon-time soap opera. Today, however, I sat in my usual chair and began to watch the television set while it was still off. I began to get fidgety and couldn't help thinking about the things that I was missing out on because of the fact that the television was turned off...This is when I realized ... I was so involved in the fictional lives of TV characters that they seemed to be part of reality to me. From then on the longer I looked at the television set, the uglier it got. I used to see it as a screen that was full of excitement and color, and now it was simply a grey box.

Teresa: When I had to sit and watch a TV that was not on, I felt like my best friend had died or was furiously mad at me. I could not get a response and I was furious in return. I was so frustrated that I could not write the assignment until Professor McGrane asked if anyone was angry about this. Then I realized what was wrong and what the experiment had proven. I am very dependent on TV (and I don't think of myself as a big TV watcher for lack of time) and just being in the same room with it really bothered me. I felt lonely and silly. What is shocking to me would probably be unbelievable to the average American. Our closest friend is our television.

The Problem of Not Having a Problem

In our reflections on television, the very first problem to address is the problem of not having a problem, of not having any difficulty. The existing media, and commercial television in particular, are just the way they are. Period. Nothing is wrong with them. Nothing is right with them. They *just* are. When anything just is, it has achieved the status of a natural reality, a piece of nature. It has transcended the human realm of the accomplished. To be accomplished is to retain the stamp of origin: "This is declared and achieved into being and it could have been different than it is." It is one possible way among others. It doesn't *have to* be that way. There is no *necessity* in its existence but rather accomplishment in its existence. If it has been brought into existence, it is transparent that it can be altered, changed, or taken back out of existence. To ask of a social institution, "Can we envision it otherwise?" is an invitation to think differently. To issue an invitation to think differently *is already* thinking differently. It is thinking that is not completely and unconsciously submissive to the status quo.

Can we see a problem with the existing media? If we *can't* get access to seeing the existing media as problematic, if for us they "just are," we can't get access to the sociological imagination in this arena. From the perspective of critical sociology, of thinking committed to the freedom and power of thinking, and of thinking committed to the freedom and power of human liberation and transformation, we are in "denial." We are in denial of the realm of possibility, and we have collapsed the possible into the realm of the already existing. By way of refinement and qualification, we also want to say here that having a strong relationship with reality doesn't make impossible the realm of possibility. Having a robust relationship with reality, acknowledging the truth of existing social situations, is not the same as "adjusting oneself to reality" or to the existence of the status quo, the existing institutional arrangements of our media. To say, "That's just how things are" is, we hold, the voice of cynicism and resignationism. On the other hand, "I refuse to accept how things are" is often the voice of rebellion in the negative, adolescent sense of "mere rebellion," of "wishful thinking." This is quite different from "I accept and acknowledge how things are but that doesn't mean I approve of it" and it doesn't mean "I can't see a radical transformation of it." Acceptance is not the same as approval or endorsement or justification.

The point is not to criticize television. That would really only add further to the television culture. To criticize is insufficient and even counter-productive. Usually to criticize a social institution really only reinforces it into further existence. To become aware of television is more to the point.

Is it Possible to Observe Television Today?

The way we see television is never what we see on the television. The nature of the medium requires us to look through it, like the car windshield while we are driving down the highway. To look *at* it alters the very nature and structure of the experience. To look *at* TV alters the whole emotional context of the experience. It's a little like going from the semi-hypnotic, longing, loving, mesmerizing gaze into your beloved's beautiful eyes, where you are sort of lost, swimming and swooning in their beauty, over to the ophthalmologists scrutinizing gaze, the gaze that sees into the form, structure, and functioning of a patient's eyeball.

In the process of examining TV, we are also examining the belief system and the socially constructed reality in which we live. The real difficulty in addressing the presence and the problem of the media is to articulate what the real problem *is*. The challenge lies in finding a space from which to ask questions and a platform to launch an analysis. If you're a fish in the ocean, how do you stop breathing the water in and out long enough to be able to get enough distance from it so as to notice it? So, initially, let's oversimplify: Let's say that the electronic media *as* the all-encompassing environment, *as* the all-pervading network and the matrix of our thoughts, *is* the problem.

As we mentioned earlier, this is deeply analogous to the problem of questioning, studying, and becoming aware of the presence of language. Any attempt to become aware of the presence of language is itself already deeply compromised, implicated, and "contaminated" as it were by the back-door presence of language in the very attempt to become aware of it in the first place. McLuhan insists that all media involve some form of transcendence and some form of bewitchment such that whatever medium we are exposed to is the one we cannot see. Let's consider the question "*Is it possible to observe TV?*" next to the question "*Is it possible to observe the words in a book?*" Let us return for a moment to our earlier remarks about becoming aware of the medium of print. Let us look at reading as a socially acquired practice. When we examine reading from a phenomenological perspective, a certain instant transcendence becomes palpably visible. To say that "We read the words on the page" really passes over an astonishing world of accomplishments. *To "see" the words on the page, we must first stop "reading" the words on the page.*

The twentieth-century German playwright, Bertolt Brecht, invented the "alienated moment" technique whereby the actor on stage in the middle of his drama abruptly "breaks character" and turns literally and directly to the audience for a moment to make a comment—then she or he "goes back" into character and into the drama. If you will indulge us in a Brechtian moment, please just stop reading this sentence/book for a moment and try to become aware of it as black markings on a white page.... If we are seeing the ink markings, we are not reading. When we are seeing, we are observing a mark, a thing on the page—sort of like a smudge of ink on the page—then we are seeing a thing-in-the-world. To read the page is to *not see it as* a thing in the world. The practice of reading is always an accomplishment of transcendence, a going beyond what is immediately and sensibly there. To "see" the words on the page would be like "hearing" the sounds coming out of your friends' mouths when they are speaking to you. You can't hear the sounds once you have "learned" the language. In calligraphy—etymologically "beautiful"(calli) "writing"(graphy)—you draw or paint letters, and each letter is a one-of-a-kind beautiful representation, an art work. Mechanical typography in a mass-produced book alters that. You can somewhat see calligraphy, especially Chinese, Tibetan, Sanskrit, but you have a very difficult time seeing the alphabet, the actual choreographed script of the typographical alphabet. You can somewhat "hear" the sounds of a foreign language being spoken in your presence but it's almost impossible to hear the sounds of your native English language being spoken. To attempt to do that, to make the familiar, once again, strange you must interrupt the flow, fracture the familiar. You must put the brakes on of ordinary, ongoing, active interpretation. You must brake with the magic, magnetic pull of accomplishing ordinary reality.

To read is to not see. It is to pass beyond the seen to the intended. To watch television is to not see; it is to pass beyond the visible, the actual, to the intended, to the narrative, the story. If the page is empty, you can't read it. If it is filled with a heap of letters all thrown together helter-skelter, you can't read it. If it is Standard English, in standard sentences, you can read it. *You can read it, but now you can't see it.* That is to say you can't read it and see it simultaneously. You must, with great effort, resist reading it to see it. You need the ink marks there on the page to go beyond the ink marks there on the page into the words and meanings. You need the sounds coming out of someone's mouth to understand what he or she is saying, but you must travel right past the sounds even as you register and hear them to the meaning. It is with immense difficulty that you can dis-attend to the meaning of someone's words and attend alone to the sounds of their words.

We are directly in the presence of transcendence, of going beyond, when we are reading. We must both touch upon and fly past the actual marks on the page to somehow accomplish the extraordinary yet ordinary miracle of reading. Likewise with TV, we touch upon and fly past the framed shot to co-create the "story." If we dwell too attentively or too inertly upon the sign itself, we cease to be engaged in reading, in TV-ing. We drop back underneath the game of activity, of actively engaging in the meaning-making story, of the narrative. We plummet right underneath the great highway of movement, speed, direction, and doing and find ourselves in the presence of the material, thing-like gravel that makes up the highway.

To notice and transcend, to notice and shoot by, seems to be an essential phenomenological structure that we practice when we do reading and when we do tv-ing. It would seem that the dog, or cat, that the animal consciousness doesn't do this, doesn't engage in this accomplishment. The animal focuses on the finger that is pointing at the moon. It does not notice, read, and transcend the pointing finger toward the moon. It does not read in the way we do. As we are here addressing this phenomenon, "intentionality" and "transcendence" are not part of animal being. Similarly with "reading" television, the animal and the infant see the finger and remain with it. It takes much work, training, and development for us to learn to read/view the TV. We notice the still photo, the scene, the camera depicting what's in front of it, but then we instantaneously transcend that to the story, the drama, the show, the meaning. When you read, you are dwelling in the space of meaning. You are in reading-land. When you watch TV, you are in TV-land, media land. You are not totally in the sensuous world, the material world. You transcend the material world into the symbolic world, the mediated world of meaning, of intention, of story. You are in the astonishing world of thought and imagination. What extraordinary magic is this ordinary, incantatory practice of reading words and watching television!

The Technical Events Test and the Media Consensus Trance

The number of technical events counted by students in a 10-minute period typically ran from 90+ to more than 350. The most extraordinary thing about this aspect of the experiment was that *almost none of us had actually noticed these events or their frequency before.* What does this tell us? We've all been in our media-created Platonic Caves, our Matrixes, watching television for years and yet have never actually *seen* it.

If we may, we'd like to put in a word here regarding our reader's desire to simply *imagine* our exercises in media de-socialization rather than actually *do* them. If we said to you to *imagine* how many technical events you would count in 10 minutes of watching television, all you would get really is the speculations of your own socialized imagination. Imagination, speculation, common sense, won't help us much here in our study of media, self, and society. We have to actually *do* the experimental exercises and have the experience. There is no replacement for the experience of doing the exercises.

Tom: Doing the TET automatically takes away the unconscious absorption; it takes the illusion of reality out of the show. And then you realize that the narrative element is the missing link: it connects the jumble of pictures and technical events together into one coherent smooth flowing object. Not until you actually do the TET do you realize that it all comes in bits and pieces.

Joanna: The technical events counting blew me away. Counting these technical events also made me tired. The speed of the activity made my head spin. I started to get nervous. I was beginning to lose control, writing in almost a frenzy. I felt sorry for my eyes and my poor brain that I had subjected to this chaos. I started to become annoyed! I wanted to scream, "STOP, ALREADY!" I ended up throwing my notebook and pen at the set, snorting obscenities all the while.

Jon: I sat down in front of my TV to do this experiment. I was going to mark down every time a technical event occurred. I then realized that this was the first time in my entire life when I was going to pay attention to something other than the content of the show I was watching. What I mean is that as I started counting the technical events the content of the show was meaningless. When I did this I had the set muted. When I turned on the sound I found it increasingly difficult not to pay attention to what was going on in the story of the show. I would lose count because I would be distracted by the show.

As we've mentioned, McLuhan held that whatever medium we are exposed to is the one we ignore. While we are watching TV, the last thing that we can SEE is TV. Immersion in the message prevents us from seeing the medium. We can't simultaneously do both. *Watching TV prevents us from observing TV.*

As a social business institution, our television media is designed to accomplish two things: to hypnotize and to sell. The zombie consumer is the order of the day. It does this by brilliant technical wizardry, not by the substance of its content.

What needs to be highlighted is the awesome yet ordinary and familiar experience that when we turn on TV, we get in some fashion *switched unconscious.*

Miles: My brother, when we were both younger, used to trick me out of my chair in front of the TV. He would wait for the most opportune moment and then he would strike. While I was engrossed in a particular show he would come over and tap me on the shoulder. With a medium tone of voice he'd tell me to get out of HIS chair. Of course I would be so mesmerized by the TV show I could only comprehend a little of what he was saying. All I could think of was someone was tapping me on the shoulder and interrupting my show! I would become so frustrated I would move not even aware that he had just taken my seat, the one I had sat in the whole night. Not aware, that is, until the commercial, then I could think straight again. I think that says it all. When the television is on, people turn into vegetables in front of it...TV commands or demands your attention. It sucks all of your creative juices from you and leaves you nothing. I am now aware of the trance like state I am in. There's an imaginary beam of light coming out of the TV set holding my line of sight rigidly in place, staring straight at the TV. It's rather like highway hypnosis. You just sit watching.

The whole culture of watching, the "*Society of the Spectacle*" in Guy DeBrod's (1967) chthonic analysis, promotes and reinforces a machinery of unconsciousness, wherein we begin living more and more on a hazy background of enchantment and mesmerism. In uncovering and examining the media-impregnated quality of consciousness, we confront that disturbing phenomenon that Charles Tart has called the "consensus trance." What we are experiencing here is a media-induced consensus trance, a brain-fade. There is also operative here a sort of retroactive reevaluation of our past relationship to television-land. Through our Un-TV experiment, we discovered that long ago we became bewitched by TV. This Sleeping Beauty- or Matrix-type experience of awakening and discovering the media consensus trance can be vivid, shocking, and alarming.

> *Terry:* After noting all the technical events on television in ten minutes I came away shocked. As I tried to count all the special effects used on programs, news, and commercials I found it rather difficult to keep count. There was approximately one technical event every second. Most of the special effects were comprised of camera focusing, as well as words flashed on the screen, scenery changes, mood changes, geography changes, and other changes that seemed to be everyday occurrences, but not so ordinary except on TV. How often does one encounter flashes of imagery every millisecond, where the images have no continuity with the whole scheme of reality in the span of five minutes? The only place that might resemble such imagery is deep in our subconscious, where the mind is constantly flashing pictures which we call memory. This leads me to wonder if television affects us more than we might admit. These subtle imageries come so fast that we do not consciously pick them up, but unfortunately, our subconscious does. Maybe that is why commercials are so effective in controlling desires.

Our very strong wide-eyed and squinting spectatorship muscles have been developed by watching TV—by watching the shadows on the cave wall—for many, many years. In this critical, Un-TV, experimental approach, the familiar spectatorship muscles weaken somewhat, and the unfamiliar engagement and awareness muscles may kick in. We may become aware that *developing the powers of observation and the powers of awareness is very distinct from developing the powers of spectatorship.*

Deeply engaging in the technical events test personally, each of us had a disturbing realization: *We began to see how much we have not seen.* We also began to see the illusory character of so much of what we have seen—seen and taken to be rock-real. This realization, we believe, came about through changing the orientation of our mind. The orientation was changed from being absorbed by the content, the story, of the media to paying attention to the medium itself, and by extension, from being absorbed by the contents of our experience to paying attention to the process of experience itself.

Labor in the Mode of Relaxation

Bruce: What a game, Dodgers ahead by two in the third inning. Oh, I'd better do my experiment 1,2,3,4, 196,197,198! OK ... What happened? I have no clue what the score is or for that matter who is up. TV is a vastly complicated maze of technical events dubbed into a background. I have no idea how we can look right through all of this to make sense of a show. We take for granted and plainly ignore the super slo-mo, scouting reports, and the shots from the Goodrich blimp ... Ah just kidding, the Goodyear blimp. How did I know to distinguish? We go on ignorant to the manipulation of media. I find it hard to relax now that I can see the constant cutting, flashing, zooming, and interrupting. It's so confusing.

Kandi: I decided to turn the sound off and count the Technical Events and see if there was a difference. There was. I became suddenly very aware that this was only a show, that the characters were only acting and that everything happening was contrived. *I always knew it was a TV program but I think I pushed it into the back of my mind while I watched.* Somehow some part of me believed it was real and only by making myself look at it closely could that part see it was fake. The pictures lost all their previous meaning. I could see images but they weren't real, they were just pictures on a screen.

Technical events *produce* the illusion of being natural, realistic, and non-produced. "Reality TV" TV shows have amplified this produced illusion in ever-more-powerful ways. As Karl Marx's sustained analysis on the quasi-magical, fetishistic properties of "commodities" testified to, the process of production is *hidden* in the objects of production. In terms of television production, a good cut is one you don't notice, as the television editors say. Engaging in the technical events test, we realize that watching a show is *not* watching actors act but watching camera tricks and sound effects transpire.

In a play, in a live theatre performance, it is the actor who is the artist in charge. It is the actor who is making creative artistic choices. Live theatre is the actor's medium; in television (and film), the director or editor is the artist in charge. With TV, the *method* of presentation is 100 times richer and more complex than the *matter* being presented. The viewer isn't watching the actor, the human dimension, but visually tracking the magical effects of graphic and image technology at work. The viewer comes to deeply identify, as Walter Benjamin noted, *not with the character but rather with the camera*, hence the overwhelming voyeuristic quality of television, hence the "society of the spectacle."

We all have a general sense of how much work goes into the television we see. We have almost no sense of how much work goes into the seeing of television. The practice of watching TV is a highly complex achievement that, once achieved, we accomplish unconsciously, without awareness. It has become as easy and as second nature as walking (which itself is a remarkable accomplishment—watch any toddler trying to learn).

> *Alfonso:*   I began to realize that the media is with me always. Throughout the years I have been a student of the media from an infant age where I could consciously notice technical events, to an age where I no longer see them unless I am forced by a homework assignment to intentionally look for them.

There is an extraordinarily artificial feeling of naturalness and spontaneity happening here. We are unaware that the practice of "watching TV" is a practice. We have never experienced the practice of "watching TV" *as a phenomenon in its own right*. As McLuhan says,

> The transforming power of media is easy to explain, but the ignoring of this power is not at all easy to explain. It goes without saying that the universal ignoring of the psychic action of technology bespeaks some inherent function, some essential numbing of consciousness such as occurs under stress or shock conditions.
>
> (McLuhan 1964:265)

One of our students captured well the stress conditions being produced while watching TV:

> *Tim:*   I was astounded at the number of technical events which exist during the course of a television program that my conscious mind ignores.

It was amazing that the multitudes of these events go unnoticed by my seemingly trained mind, while my subconscious mind is bombarded with literally thousands of technical events each day of viewing. During the course of a cop show, I counted nearly 200 technical events within the ten minute interval. To convince myself that this was not simply a result of the unique style of this show's directing, I switched to an old rerun of Dallas and was amazed to count nearly 175 events. Although these numbers seem high, the actual number of events is even higher for they came so quickly that I could not count them all fast enough. During the course of counting these events, I realized how abrasive TV programming must be to my subconscious mind, while it is subjected to the infinite number of focusing, refocusing, directing and redirecting that occurs during the course of every television program.

Why are we unaware of the practice as a practice? Doing the Technical Events Test almost forces us to notice that watching TV is an active, ongoing achievement that we accomplish for another first time through each routine time we sit down and do it. We see what the texture of the experience called *watching TV* consists of, and simultaneously we experience the strong shock of *seeing that we haven't seen* the texture of the experience in all these years of watching TV. This is a dramatic example of what ethnomethodologists mean when they say that social reality is actively and ongoingly constructed and accomplished and yet never consciously noticed.

The quality of this non-awareness is similar to the non-spot that Julian Jaynes discusses with regard to our physical vision and our consciousness in his controversial work, *The Origin of Consciousness in the Breakdown of the Bicameral Mind:*

> We are conscious less of the time than we think, because we cannot be conscious of when we are not conscious...There is a way to point this out. If you close your left eye and stare at the left margin of this page, you are not at all conscious of a large gap in your vision about four inches to the right. But, still staring with your right eye only, take your finger and move it along a line of print from the left margin to the right, and you will see the top of it disappear into this gap and then reappear on the other side This is due to a two-millimeter gap on the nasal side of the retina where the optic nerve fibers are gathered together and leave the

eye for the brain. The interesting thing about this gap is that it is not so much a blind spot as it is usually called; it is a non-spot. A blind man sees his darkness. But you cannot see any gap in your vision at all, let alone be conscious of it in any way. Just as the space around the blind spots is joined without any gap at all, so consciousness knits itself over its time gaps and gives the illusion of continuity.

(Jaynes 1976:24–25)

Through becoming aware of how we rapidly crochet and integrate discrete scenes, we also became aware that we had all along been doing this integration without awareness and without noticing that we were doing it. We had all along produced the illusion of continuity.

TV and Boredom

One slight variation on this experiment that we tried was to have students *compare* watching TV for 15 minutes without turning it on with watching a tree for 15 minutes.

Becky: By observing a television for fifteen minutes, I learned absolutely nothing. In fact, I was so bored I kept looking at my timer and gave up after four minutes. I was nervous, bored, and uncomfortable. How, then, can I watch television for hours upon end and not be bored? Is it really that entertaining? I do not think so. It is the hypnotic factor that television has, and yet after hours of watching I do not feel fulfilled. When I observed a tree, however, I was startled when my timer went off. I was not bored; I was intrigued by the movement and more in tune with every aspect of the tree. Both the tree and the television are inanimate objects, and yet both made me feel completely different. I wanted more from the television, and yet got more from looking at the tree.

The average American watches four hours of television a day. In the context of our experimental exercise of watching TV for 15 minutes without turning it on and of counting the number of technical events for 10 minutes, a question often arises: *Why don't we get bored?* How can most of us stare at a box emitting light for hours on end and not experience boredom? Perhaps we do experience boredom but it gets covered over and camouflaged with mental speed.

Armine: I found it very startling that in a five minute period I had experienced 120 technical events. I don't think I have ever noticed what an astronomical amount of input my brain was receiving from the television. It's amazing to me that with all this activity going on people don't feel overloaded and end up with a splitting headache after watching only five minutes. After discovering how much excitement goes on in a five minute period I can't understand how so many of us can sit and passively watch television for hours at a time, especially when we just want to relax.

The slow fading-in, fading-out technique is used continually with conventional TV programs. The commercial, in contrast, doesn't fade-into the screen smoothly but rather explodes onto the screen, causing us, as a consequence, to watch this strange event as if it were an emergency. The advertisements are thus experienced as permeated with a kind of mental adrenaline and a highly subtle, sophisticated, subliminal form of visual violence. This is a violence to ordinary perception: For violence, like sex, is always attention-captivating. The living room couch now often functions as a meditation cushion in the service not of enlightenment and peace of mind but of "endarkenment" and a thrilling, benumbing, mental chaos. In *Mediated*, de Zengotita addresses the "hyperactive, rushed" quality of the media experience in somewhat similar terms:

> On some level, were rushing even when we're relaxing…Even if we're poleaxed for hours on end in front of the TV, our minds must keep pace with the hyperpacing of the ads and shows…That's why television (and movies) provides us with all those stress dramas…Actually, though, stress dramas are about the working lives of the media people who make them. This is a fundamental insight, another example of the unnoticed ways that media saturates experience…motion must be maintained.
>
> (de Zengotita 2005:192)

Counting the technical events brings about a marked shift, somewhat of a paradigm shift. When we get caught up and quasi-tranced into the story line, the technical events disappear. When, in doing this exercise, we get attentively caught up in counting the technical events, the storyline vanishes. In doing the TET, what we notice is the discrete segments of independent images that are presented with a machine gun–like rapid-fire quality. As we watch, we, the "passive" viewers, apparently put together, synthesize, and integrate the scenes: We link, we knit, we chain, we retain the past scenes and anticipate the future ones. We methodically weave them all together into a coherent narrative. A high-speed filling-in-the-blanks and connecting-the-dots occurs. Our actively synthesizing mind, our mental interpretive labor, goes on, while nevertheless being experienced in the mode of relaxation and absorption. This high-speed integration of often wildly disconnected phenomena (angles, scenes, persons, music) is experienced in the mode of blank and passive absorption. It would seem that our mind is in a whirring high gear without our knowing it. Mander addresses this pointedly:

> This difference between internally generated and imposed imagery is at the heart of whether it is accurate to say that television relaxes the mind. Relaxation implies renewal. One runs hard, then rests. While resting the muscles first experience calm and then, as new oxygen enters them, renewal. When you are watching, absorbing techno-guru, your mind may be in alpha, but it is certainly not empty mind. Images are pouring into it. Your mind is not quiet or calm or empty. It may be nearer to dead, or zombie-ized. It is occupied. No renewal can come from this condition. For renewal, the mind would have to be at rest, or once rested, it would have to be seeking new kinds of stimulation, new exercise. Television offers *neither rest nor stimulation*. Television inhibits your ability to think, but it does not lead to freedom of mind, relaxation or renewal. It leads to a more exhausted mind. You may have time out from prior obsessive thought patterns, but that's as far as television goes. The mind is never empty, the mind is filled. What's worse, it is filled with someone else's obsessive thoughts and images.
>
> (Mander 1977:213–214)

Sitting in the midst of this blizzard of technical events, *why don't we get lost or dizzy?* Counting the technical events consciously makes our mind feel like a tennis ball being rapidly bounced back and forth, ricocheting hither and yon. It painfully demonstrates how many times our mind has to readjust itself to a new scene: It is the quintessence of activity in the mode of passivity.

Sara: I saw 297 technical events! 297! I only saw about 170 the first time that we did this experiment. (My eye is becoming quick in catching any changes that take place.) During the commercials I could not count the technical events fast enough. The picture and the music were always changing so rapidly that my eyes could not keep up with all of the changes. Maybe this is one of the reasons why television is so engaging. It is stimulating. Not because of its fabulous content, but because it keeps the eyes and the mind working to keep up and connect all of the changing images…I now truly believe that *we don't watch TV solely for the interest of a program, but for the activity that our mind does as we watch it.*

Ken: My first reaction to the number of technical events (126) was, do we actually soak all this in during normal viewing? I then thought of the subliminal advertising, the actual cost of using these technical events, and decided, we absolutely do take it all in. So, if we take it all in, what is that doing to our attention span? I mean, according to the directors of these shows, we can't concentrate on one thing for more than a second or two, if that. I suppose an argument could be made that the pre-TV person already had a tiny attention span, and these directors are simply catering to our already feeble minds. But for some strange reason, I think TV is doing its best to shrink not only our attention spans but our intellect as well.

TV Without Sound: A Loud, Clamorous Silence

To see more clearly the nature and role of "technical events" in conventional television watching, it's helpful to watch the TV without sound.

Christopher: Without the sound on, it made me acutely aware of how often the scenes and camera angles changed. It made me see how separate and unrelated the actions are. The storyline tries to convey a sense of continuity to the show so that even after five minutes of commercials the show still makes some sort of sense. But when the storyline is taken away, the picture itself reveals nothing but unrelated scenes. They seem to be simply what the producers thought would be exciting to watch and a story line was fit around the action.

Tim: I hated watching my show without the sound on. I felt as if I was missing something. It was as if I was being left out of the TV world. It was an uncomfortable feeling to realize that while I watched TV normally, I feel a part of it. However, without the sound, I felt as though I could not take part in the conversation or actions of the program. In other words, I could not experience the show. I felt concerned that this feeling of rejection and loneliness could be caused by a television set. I felt as though the TV had a spell over me when I watched it normally. Now, however, without the sound, and the feeling of belonging it usually caused, the spell seemed to be broken.

As we have stressed, in counting the technical events, we as viewers are amazed at how much we fill in the gaps to co-create a story. As Charles Tart talks about a consensus-trance, so we might here talk about being caught up in a narrative-trance. We have been programmed to become narrative-subjects by being continuously subjected to the developmental narrative mode. Our eyes do not see what is actually there because our narrative-trained mind overrides our eyes. We don't see with our eyes, we see with our programming, and we are programmed to see programs (stories, narratives). TV programs us to not notice the technical events, to not notice the details, to not in that sense pay attention. To watch TV programs is to become programmed. The TV is a programming device, not a communicating device. It's not communicating, it's programming. We do not perceive/experience the TV as a device, which it is, but as a reality, which it is not.

Cairn: Here are some of the things I saw: some mothers, when they do laundry, have lucky lightning bolts strike their clothes. A woman with little-girl pigtails wearing a football jersey only uses the weight room to get a guy—not to use the weights. Some airplanes can fly two ways at once—coming and going. Yogurt makes people happy. No one on television has feet. When people convene, they always invite odd numbers of people; most humans live in groups of three. People don't talk to each other; they face the viewer when they speak. Many times the camera set me right behind someone's shoulder, and made me look over. I felt very voyeuristic. I also became increasingly frustrated as I watched. Nothing stays steady. In five minutes' time, the camera switched angles 53 times.

During the news program, the camera stayed steadier, but the show did include the same elements of entertainment—all the interviewers acted emotionally. However, one man and one woman remained serious throughout. They didn't notice when the sign changed behind their heads, and they didn't change clothes between shots, like the other actors in the entertainment program did. The news section that I saw showed pictures of hospitals, factories, graphs, and people winning lotteries—no sign of government. Also, if I hadn't been "trained" by experience to recognize advertisements, I couldn't tell when the news stopped and the commercial began. There were no borders between the different types of programming.

In discussing this explicit "lack of borders" between the different types of programming called "show" versus "commercial," another student related how she once had a foreign visitor from a very remote region of the world staying at her home. This visitor had never seen television before, and became completely confused while they were watching. At one moment, he was seeing a family scene unfold in a living room; then, suddenly, other people were playing volleyball on a beach while drinking Pepsi-Cola. While he was trying to relate this scene to the family in their living room, suddenly he was looking down from above at an airplane flying through the sky; he thought for a moment he saw the family's mother serving drinks inside the airplane, but at the next moment she was back with her husband and children. Then, suddenly, they were driving down the street in an automobile and were no longer in their living room. The student said the visitor became quite upset and disoriented. Perhaps TV should come with a surgeon general's stamp to all human beings who are about to be exposed to it for the first time, "Warning: TV may be harmful to your relationship to reality."

TV as reality, as a place where we live, and as a critical instrument in the social construction of reality are themes we more closely examine in the next chapter.

3

REALITY TV

TV is a Place Where We Live

Every person in our time lives in two worlds. One is the natural, flesh-and-blood world that has been the environment of human beings since the origins of Homo sapiens…The other world in which most human beings live today is the mass media world.

(Bagdikian 2005:xii)

Perhaps it's not TV per se, but rather that TV's boundaries with the world are both fuzzy and acid-like. It's an object in the world, yet it is *boundary dissolving* in such a way that we easily succumb to experiencing it as accessing the world. "It is easy to overlook a deceptively simple fact: one is always *watching television* when one is watching television rather than having any other experience" (Winn 2002:3). We seem to fall into intractable psychic confusion over what is world experience and what is TV experience. Bill McKibben did a bizarre and immensely revealing experiment wherein he taped and watched everything on TV in the United States during a 24 hour period—more than 400 channels, network, and cable. He then compared point by point what he had learned in that endless day of TV—it took him four months—with what he learned in a 24-hour period camping out in the wilderness. He wrote of his discoveries in his *The Age of Missing Information* (1992):

If my endless day of television reminded me of anything, it's that electronic media have become an environment of their own—that to the list of neighborhood and region and continent and planet we must now add television as *a place where we live*. And the problem is not that it exists—the problem is that it supplants. Its simplicity makes complexities hard to fathom.

(McKibben 1992:53; emphasis added)

We contend that a person who constantly practices the electronic confusion of these two experiences can lose the ability to distinguish fantasy from reality. And, of course, this is not only an individual phenomenon but a collective one as well in that constantly and effortlessly traveling back and forth between these two worlds *an entire culture will lose the ability to realize it has lost the ability to distinguish fantasy from reality.*

The Electronic Plug-in Drug

TV is a mind-altering experience. With our Un-TV exercises, we have endeavored to highlight the shift on our sense of reality that the practice of watching television can induce in us. Perhaps the closest analogue to this phenomenon is our contemporary notion of "drugs"—a highly addictive, mind-altering substance that affects our perception of reality.

Chris I've discovered TV to be a powerful addicting drug of not thinking, at least not your own thoughts. I don't think there has ever been such a drug so widely used by the populace, and so mentally harmful. Harmful in a way that it stops all one's individual mental thoughts. When I watched TV, with or without the sound on, I did not think. When I began to watch it, all of my thoughts completely vanished, and I sat there watching a story. And the story was all that I was. Of course extraneous thoughts entered my mind, but these were simple, quick, one-sentence thoughts without any further thought or elaborations. The thought of a newly developing relationship of mine popped into my mind for five seconds, and then it was gone, forgotten, as the TV resumed occupying my entire mind. However, yesterday I had spent three hours thinking and writing a letter about my thoughts to her. Every other thought of my own, not the TV's, that also came to mind only stayed there for a couple of seconds, until the TV took over my mind and relieved me with an empty mind. In a way, TV has trained me to watch TV. Every scene, camera shot, or news clip is based on quick, short, story thoughts that pass by and keep moving so quickly that you have no time to think further about them … because instantly you're presented with another entertaining, thought controlling shot.

TV is an electronic drug that aggravates in the long run the problem it temporarily assuages in the short run, and we can see at this stage that "drug" is more a literal rather than metaphorical term. Listen to the precise qualities present in an electronic drug-game experience for the compulsive, addicted gambler as described in one of the most well-known textbooks on psychoactive drug addiction, *Uppers, Downers, All Arounders—Physical and Mental Effects of Psychoactive Substances*:

> There are some things that make some games more potent and more powerful than others according to Robert Hunter, an expert in the field of pathological gambling….For the 5% who are pathological gamblers what makes a game exciting for the average person makes it deadly for them: … the ability to lose yourself in the game, to block out external stimuli, to get lost and focus solely on what's in front of you …
>
> (Inaba and Cohen 2005:XX)

This double-barrel effect of simultaneously devastating while becalming the addict is also powerfully present in the ordinary television experience.

> *Sara:* Soon I stopped thinking about the TV and I began thinking about myself and all of my problems and all of the things I had to do. Then it dawned on me that no wonder TV is so addictive, it keeps me from having to think about my life. It is a form of drug. But like any drug the problem is that it makes one's ability to cope with problems much more difficult. If I watch it to keep myself from thinking about my problems, it doesn't mean my problems are not there. It means that I am not coping with them.

Predator 3: Watch a Watcher

In classical Greek lore, one of the three Gorgons was named Medusa: If you gazed at her even for just an instant, you were turned to stone. The practice, habit, and accomplishment of watching TV is our modern, electronic version of Medusa.

At this point, we should also look at the results from the segment of the Un-TV experiment that asked students to watch not TV but someone watching TV.

Mike: People are so boring when they watch TV.

Justin: While watching someone watch TV the majority of the time I felt very distant to the watcher, as if they weren't really present and in the same moment I was. They were very still, had a very slow consistent breath and their eyes remained fixed in almost the same position for the entire ten minutes. I saw them in front of me, but in a very detached and unattached manner. I imagined that almost anything could be going on around them and their gaze would have remained fixated on the box in front of them so long as it remained on. Interestingly enough, as soon as I turned it off their entire demeanor changed in an instant. The watcher suddenly became active and energetic, eyes darting every which way in search of the culprit who turned off their amusement. Indeed, once this happened I actually felt the aura of the watcher as a real human before me and not just their physical presence. While watching TV they were nothing but a shell, but when TV was removed they instantaneously became full of life.

At the end of their 10-minute observation period of "watching a TV watcher," students were instructed to go up to the TV with as neutral a manner as possible and, simply, turn it off. They were then to observe—with as much of a beginner's mind as they could call forth—what happened.

Being mesmerized by what's happening on TV is something you can more or less vaguely feel happening to yourself; but when you watch someone watching TV, you see perhaps more vividly what's actually happening to you when you're watching TV. This is a little like the difference between trying to observe yourself being affected while drinking a half bottle of vodka and watching, coldly sober, someone else become affected while drinking a half bottle. In *The Plug-In Drug*, Marie Winn says, "just as alcoholics are only vaguely aware of their addiction, feeling that they control their drinking more than they really do ('I can cut it out any time I want—I just like to have three or four drinks before dinner') many people overestimate their control over television watching." (Winn 2002: 32).

Alec: I noticed that the person went into a trance. While he was staring at this box nothing seemed to bother him. His TV seemed to take him into another world which he seemed to belong to. Then when I turned it off it was like when a person is under a trance and a finger is snapped to make them come out. He looked at me like I was crazy and told me to turn it back on. I realized TV is kind of like a high, you never want it to go away, especially when you're in the middle of it…Now the television kind of scares me.

Nicole: An important background note is that my father did not grow up with a television set because he was raised in a very poor family in Morocco. My mother had a television in her house from the age of five on…As I watched the two of them, the differences in their viewing styles soon became apparent. While my mother sat fairly still, with her eyes perfectly still and transfixed on the screen, my dad fidgeted… but perhaps most interesting, as he watched I noticed that his irises were constantly in motion. I think my mother's watching behavior is probably more typical…this led me to hypothesize that perhaps only by watching television during childhood can you learn how to watch properly. My father having never watched television until he was a teenager simply doesn't know the right way to watch. That ability to enter an altered state of consciousness during television watching may be, like sight itself, one that can only be acquired early in life. My father missed that window of opportunity, and so, although he certainly enjoys watching television more than my mother does, he doesn't watch in the same focused way.

As we mentioned earlier, when we are in that "zone," it's almost as if we do not know which world we live in, the one that we exist in or the one that TV creates. Philip K. Dick's science fiction novel, *The Man in the High Castle*, describes a historically alternative world in which WW II had been won by the Third Reich. The Nazi occupation authorities legalize a specific drug to pacify the occupied population in a way very similar to that the citizens of Huxley's *Brave New World* are given the drug "soma." Terence McKenna, in his work, *Food of the Gods*, slightly alters the drug Dick envisioned that the Nazi occupation authorities used:

> The drug was the first of a growing group of high-technology drugs that deliver the user into an alternative reality by acting directly on the user's sensorium, without chemicals being introduced into the nervous system. It was television. No epidemic or addictive craze or religious hysteria has ever moved faster or made as many converts in so short a time...no drug in history has so quickly or completely isolated the entire culture of its users from contact with reality. And no drug in history has so completely succeeded in remaking in its own image the values of the culture that it has infected.
>
> (McKenna 1992:218)

McKenna sees that the effects on our collective consciousness that television creates has allowed the media to force-feed us the values of the culture of TV, and they have become incorporated into our own cultural values. The celebrity media culture that has been created is so deeply ingrained in our minds that we now echo its desires and are enthralled by the latest fashion, trend, or gossip that is fed to us.

TV, Live and in the Box

> *Lisa:*   As I watched the show being taped, I kept saying to myself, "This is not what I saw." Seeing it taped and watching it on television are two different things.

Glamour! Fame! Celebrity! Doesn't everyone wish they were on TV? TV is magic and, like any magic show, it's not quite the same when you know how all the magic tricks actually get accomplished. The university we teach at isn't too far from Hollywood and, for a number of years, we've been requiring students in our media classes to attend the taping of a TV show. We called this exercise "live TV?" This exercise had three parts: First they watch an episode of the show we've gotten tickets for on television, then they attend a taping of that show, then they watch that particular taping when it airs on TV.

Through direct personal experience of the actual making of a TV show, we can acquire a deeper, more genuine media literacy. Like Dorothy in *The Wizard of Oz* and Truman in *The Truman Show*, we can see what's illusion and what's the reality behind the illusion.

Robin: I was disappointed in watching the taping because it took the dream of being a glamorous movie star in a famous TV show and turned it all into a huge process of production.

Stephanie: I watched the taping of the show I saw in person and was shocked at what I felt. I had more fun watching the TV version than I did the taping! The taping was always delayed by errors or mistakes and watching the show on television, I did not have those interruptions. The show had more of an impact AS TELEVISION and I am not sure why. I felt it was funnier on television. It was weird because I never thought that anything could top seeing a show in person. In doing so, though, something is removed from the show. At least if you don't see the taping you won't be cheated when you see it on television. You won't feel like the show is not real when you see it on television.

It would seem that watching a show live makes the whole experience of TV go flat. The depth of the disillusionment expressed in the foregoing reflections is both poignant and telling. It has the poignancy of a small child discovering that her mother and father are fakes, imitations, Stepford-robot parents. Yet the worst of this Hollywood/ TV/glamour mind impoverishment that is so deeply ingrained in our culture is *that there is no sense of impoverishment*. Television culture trains us to become deeply shallow and want to be what we watch on TV.

Spectator vs Voyeur: The Dynamics of "Reality TV"

...we might say that the self-proliferating voyeuristic drive enacted by the cast members [of *Temptation Island*] in watching video clips of their partner's dates revolves around the vortex of the audience gaze— for which the entire spectacle is staged. The ostensible goal of each cast members' voyeurism is, precisely to see from the position of the Other/

audience...Thus *Temptation Island* neatly highlights...the socially complicit role played by the voyeurism of the audience.

(Andrejevic 2004:185)

What are the dynamics of voyeurism? What are the dynamics of spectatorship? What are the dynamics of television? If we combine television and voyeurism, we get televoyeurism. Lacan's enigmatic contention that in voyeurism, "What one looks at is what cannot be seen" (Andrejevic 2004:182) is crucial here. TV is the industry of voyeurism, ordinary, legitimated voyeurism.

Becoming a celebrity and watching others are the key dimensions of "reality TV." With commercial television in general, there is, we might say, the celebrity side of the screen and the anonymous viewer side of the screen. Each side depends completely on the other for its current existence. Consider the phenomena of scopophilia—the love of watching—and of voyeurism.

> Reality shows and amateur video shows dominate TV programming. It is the age of scopophilia, voyeurism, and vicarious living ... We like to watch. It is a surveillance culture.—From James Cameron's screenplay for the movie *Strange Days*.

(Andrejevic 2004:7)

The power and dynamics of voyeurism live in seeing without ourselves being seen—of being invisible while attached to watching the visible. As voyeur, we aspire to an invisible visibility. As voyeur, we are palpably invisible, an omniscient all-gazing eye that sees without itself ever being seen. There is no risk of visibility, of being seen—no risk of the vulnerability of interaction. If living interaction is the medium of human social life, watching TV is the spectacle-ization of that social, interactional life. Umberto Eco has called it the "frantic desire for the almost real" (Eco 1990:18).

From this perspective in the televisual cave, we negate and transcend actual interaction by *watching interaction*, by transforming it into being something to watch, to look at, to follow. The novelist David Foster Wallace captures quite well this peculiar voyeuristic re-enforcement of isolation and loneliness together with the transformation of this isolated loneliness into "audience-ness":

The second great-seeming thing is that television looks to be an absolute godsend for a human subspecies that loves to watch people but hates to be watched itself. For the television screen affords access only one-way. A psychic ball-check valve. We can see Them; They can't see Us. We can relax, unobserved, as we ogle. I happen to believe this is why television also appeals so much to lonely people. To voluntary shut-ins. Every lonely human I know watches way more than the average U.S. six hours a day. The lonely, like the fictive, love one-way watching.

Lonely people tend, rather, to be lonely because they decline to bear the psychic costs of being around other humans. They are allergic to people. People affect them too strongly.

But lonely people, at home, alone, still crave sights and scenes, company. Hence television. Joe can stare at Them on the screen; They remain blind to Joe. It's almost like voyeurism.

(Wallace 1997: 22–23)

With regard to watching TV, as we have mentioned, we identify with the camera. We become camera-like: watching, registering, capturing— the omniscient fly-on-the-wall syndrome. We see it all. We are in a superior, god-like deified position in regard to the people whom we are watching. Occurring here is a complete and total surveillance, an "all knowing" without it being known that we are knowing. *We are hidden from the world we are so avidly watching.*

In the conventional real world experience of voyeurism, "they" don't know that we are watching them. If they knew that we were watching, we wouldn't be in the mode of the voyeur. Their knowing that we are watching is a mode of interaction, of relationship. *The suspension of the dynamics of relationship, of the dynamics of interactional constraints, is constitutive of the very nature of watching the spectacle of TV.* Yet, paradoxically, we still feel deeply connected to the people we watch to such an extent that we feel we know them and have a relationship with them.

Of course, as David Foster Wallace observes, the media actors, whether they are trained actors or reality TV show participants, are in fact highly aware of the camera bearing down upon them. Their job as media actors is to *pretend* they are unaware, to *act as if they are not acting for the camera, to act as if there is no camera there*, to act as if they are acting as they are acting because that is how they act. As actors we forget ourselves into the scene and thereby forget the camera bearing down upon us. As audience we also forget the camera and lose ourselves into the scene that is unfolding. *We forget the camera as actors; we forget the camera as audience.* In this sense, the foundation of watching television is *forgetting the self and forgetting the camera.* As spectator, we forget our self by losing our self into the spectacle framed and produced by the camera.

Suppose we watch a voyeur on television. We watch them watch someone. We watch them watching. Do we see *our* part in all this? No. We can't see our self watching them watching. We can only see them watching. If we try to see our self see them, we collapse the television mirage circuit. We become aware of watching television, aware of our part, our participation. It is constitutive of the practice of television in our contemporary commercial media era that we forget ourselves into the show, into the circuitry of watching. We need to lose our self *into* the show to watch the show and not tumble abrasively into a critical analysis consciousness, an awareness of the self-reflective relationship of watching. Suppose in every TV scene we watch we had a back drop of a mirror continuously revealing the *presence of the camera* to us, the viewer-voyeurs. This would generate a feedback loop of continuous awareness that we are watching a staged production, that what is going on has no reason for existence other than the fact that it is being watched going on.

"At Least It Isn't Me" and Reality TV

We believe the voyeuristic enterprise of Reality TV has a deeper psychological root that explains some of its attraction. Not only does the rush of the taboo/pleasure/guilt of the voyeuristic experience of TV make Reality TV so appealing and compelling but there is a darker and baser element at work in this particular part of the medium. In watching the often degrading and exploitive experiences that most of these contestants go through, we can sit in our own homes and feel better about ourselves and say, "At least that isn't me.'

Life can't be as bad as it seems if you can see people worse off than you every day in sometimes shockingly intimate portraits. It is not the same as seeing a homeless person on the way to work or school and realizing you are better off than they are. It is getting a glimpse at the thought process and foibles of other humans in a way usually reserved for people you know intimately and personally. This permits us to be judge and jury of these individuals and in doing so somehow feel better about where we are in life.

Some of the draw of the enterprise of Reality TV then seems to be that it mediates against our own self-loathing, or at least our doubts and insecurities. Reality TV allows us to use other individual's misfortune to increase our own self-esteem. Middle school children have made this deflection process a brutal rite of passage wherein individuals cling to cliques and peer groups to avoid being targeted for ridicule. It isn't just "mean girls" at schools who partake in this venture, although some like de Zengotita would argue the adolescent female population has set a high bar in this avenue, it is a culture of put-downs that target almost anyone on the outside. Even though most middle school children know it is not right to pick on other people, "it is better someone else than me" is an easy and safer way to justify their actions and join in. Whether this is conscious or unconscious, being a part of this deflection of negativity from themselves allows their fragile sense of self to maintain some protection.

Reality TV has given adults the opportunity to continue this selfish and cruel rite of passage without fear of repercussions and to feel better about themselves in the process. We can see the faults of others vividly displayed and make value judgments and even disparaging remarks. Doing this makes it easier to accept that we might not be where we want to be in life but at least we are not the person we are watching. We can critique and place blame and think of how differently we would react in these situations without ever having to look at our own faults and doubts. TV is often used as an escape from dealing with tough situations and, in the case of Reality TV, it can be used to mediate against our own insecurities. Just as for the middle school children, Reality TV allows us to say, "It is better them than me." Instead of hiding behind cliques, we now hide behind technology as we voyeuristically engage in criticism. We might know that we have problems, but "at least that isn't me" is a powerfully addictive psychological additive to the Reality TV mix that can permit us to justify our own actions at the expense of someone else.

Watching the folly of others is proving to be a profitable business. By sanctioning us to watch others go through humiliating and degrading experiences, some of which play on our worst personal fears, the creators of these shows have deliberately focused at some of the basest parts of human nature and made a direct hit. With this, the creators can shape our reality.

TV and the Social Construction of Reality

There is, in a certain sense, a dictatorship of television power, especially with the relatively recent merging of many media corporations into only five transnational media monopolies (Bagdikian 2005). A very small group of people control the vast majority of network and cable TV. We have found in the technical events test of our Un-TV exercise —simply counting the number of camera angle changes, cuts, zooms, sound-overs, and the like—that there are essentially three main functions of the *political institution* of television (etymologically, "far-seeing," "seeing-far"). These three functions are as follows:

1. Training us to shorten our attention span
2. Making ordinary life appear dull
3. Coercing us into its reality

Shortening attention

How does having a short attention span affect the person who has been trained to have it? What qualities does a person manifest who has a long attention span? What good does it do for a social minority to reinforce a short attention span in the social majority? (As the power and influence of TV grows, the people in control of it are shrinking in numbers. When Ban Bagdikian, the dean of media studies, first published *The Media Monopoly* in 1983, 50 corporate firms dominated American mass media. To put this in perspective, there are roughly 450,000 corporations in the U.S. economy. Bagdikian's latest edition, 2004, showed that only five multinational conglomerates now control almost the entirety of American mass media—mass media in total, not just television.) Who would possibly benefit from a large portion of the population having a short attention span? Why has so much of contemporary politics become a politics of distraction? It is not too far amiss to say that in using weapons of mass distraction in today's world of media politics, elections have been reduced to the "bread and circuses" dimension of the people. As Bagdikian has said,

> Television is the quintessential short-term medium. Like jugglers, television lives for the split second. Its relationship to viewers is measured in tiny fractions. Solemn hierarchies of men and women react to overnight program ratings with something approaching nervous breakdowns because one percentage point in ratings can mean a difference of $30 million profit a year. The result of this manic concern is to design programming that will serve the split second of attention-getting rather than the humanistic substance that will stay with the viewer; the ratings race serves the advertiser's needs, not the audience's.
>
> (Bagdikian 1990:202)

It is easier to shorten the quality of attentiveness of a person than to lengthen their attention span. It is easier to increase a person's susceptibility to distraction than to strengthen their concentration ability and their ability to calm, quiet, and still their mind of distractions. (There is an old Zen analogy regarding meditation that the way to calm, clear, and quiet the mind is similar to the way to clear a churning, agitated, muddy pool—not by action, by doing, by stirring it smooth, but by stillness, by letting it be, by letting it settle itself.) The function of TV is to create, maintain, and constantly reinforce what in the Zen tradition is often called "monkey-mind." What is the good of a jumpy, volatile, scattered, hyper-monkey-mind? *The daily creation and re-creation of this type of mind is believed to be optimal in generating the "consuming" life style.* To reinforce this type of mind helps to generate a buying mood among the audience, which is believed to generate actual buying behavior as a long-term way of life. The good life is the life of consumption—not production, not creation, not action. The good life is the life of electronic reverie, of passive watching under the illusion of imaginary action: spectating. If we treat the actual block of time for American evening TV watching from 6 or 7 PM to 11 PM, we have four to five hours a day of people watching their favorite shows while simultaneously being mesmerized into a fantasy buying mood, into fantasizing about buying things. This ongoing fantasizing about the ongoing buying of new things is the central "teaching" of TV:

> [P]eople use the consumption levels and patterns portrayed in TV advertising to *evaluate their levels of personal well-being* while those same consumption patterns are simultaneously devastating the environmental and resource base on which our future depends.
>
> (Elgin 1990:10; emphasis added)

For consumerism, it is the *act of buying* rather than the *relationship of possessing* or owning that is of crucial importance.

Ordinary Life Made Dull

Regarding the drastic transformation that TV brings about in our post-TV practice (i.e., our life outside of TV watching), Mander brings home an interesting point: "When you are watching television you are seeing images that are utterly impossible in nature. This in itself qualifies the imagery for your attention, even when the content within the image is nothing you'd otherwise care about" (Mander 1977:302). On so many levels, TV transforms the way we experience reality. Because we become so conditioned and in tune with believing what is shown on TV as real, *we become skeptical of that which we only personally experience.* Our experiences in the real world become *secondary* experiences, whereas that which is experienced through TV becomes *primary.* Like every effective, long-term, complex drug addiction, TV's primary negative power lies in disguising its primary negative power in our life. Bill McKibben also addressed this phenomenon with reference to nature programs: "Something even more insidious happens when you get most of your nature through television…the 'real' nature around you, even when it's intact, begins to seem dull" (McKibben 1992:75). One of the students in our media awareness classes captured this growing dullness succinctly.

> *Cathy:* It appears that television has made my life seem to be very slow and unexciting and television adds excitement into my life by having all this action condensed into a few seconds.

The most important message of TV is that you need TV (again, the medium is the message). One way of maintaining this is to ensure that TV programming, as our media in general, is *saturated* with fantasy violence and fantasy sex in ways that our lives are certainly not.

Ritta: The mass media of television is a very thought out, precise form of visual, and auditory stimuli that never gives us an opportunity to be bored. By having all these technical stimuli, we are mesmerized to watching not only pure television, but an entire entertainment center dedicated to keeping us glued to the set. The way sound and music is utilized in television programs, also serves to make it almost difficult to find anything other than television interesting. No wonder today's society finds reading hard and boring; there are no technical events or sound effects in reading.

Coercing Us into Reality

Lexi: I never would have noticed all the action merely passively watching TV. Generally when people watch TV they are doing just that—staring at a box full of colors and sounds. They rarely notice the details. That is why commercials, and even regular programming, now bother me. If I can barely count all of the obvious stimuli coming at me I'm sure that I cannot process it all consciously. But that is probably the point, I'm sure. I'm sure everything I see and/or hear is being processed on some level. Therefore, I believe, TV affects us much more than we realize. We think we can watch a program and pick and choose different details to either believe or reject. I'm not sure anymore that that is true. I'm afraid that much more is getting through than we can consciously control.

Our culture and education conspire to condition us to need reassurance from the media (and from science) to reinforce our actions and feelings, our own, individual perceptions. When we feel we need to seek media confirmation, we both acknowledge and assume that our personal experiences *are not qualified as reality any longer.* In 1977, Jerry Mander saw this very clearly:

Slowly I began to see how the ubiquitousness of television, combined with a general failure to understand what it did to information might affect the political work we were doing. If people were believing that an image of nature was equal to or even similar to the experience of nature, and were therefore satisfied enough with the image that they did not seek out the real experience, then nature was in a lot bigger trouble than anyone realized. Or, if people believed that images of historical events or new events were equal to the events or were even close approximations to them, then historical reality was in big trouble.

(Mander 1978:26)

We lose the drive to experience direct experience and the drive to participate in meeting reality. We no longer do, we watch, and reality is someone else's creation. As Todd Gitlin has said, it's not until an event (institution, thought, principle, movement, etc.) crosses the media threshold that it takes on a solid reality for us. Stretched out across our world is the media membrane, across the threshold of which, and *only* across whose threshold, lies legitimate, confirmed reality. Though we don't have to believe what the media tell us—in terms of our own critical skepticism and, to some degree, our access to the Internet—we can't know what they don't tell us.

Television news is, in essence, entertainment-in-the-mode-of-information. News is organized, produced, presented, and packaged as if it were a game. Segments last one to two minutes and bounce from newscaster to newscaster like a basketball passed on the court (Parenti 1986:53–59). The format of the shows is completely standardized and routinized: news bits, sports bits, spontaneous kibitzing or questioning between newscasters, weather bits, and end with a human interest bit. In a very real sense, the newscasters are no more real than the characters on other entertainment shows. One sustained look reveals how much of a product and a character the newscaster is. The appearance of the newscasters—their presence as well as their looks—becomes just as vital as the news itself. They often look like mannequins and are somehow qualified to give us news by virtue of their perfect features. Whatever their actual journalistic skills, they tend to become actors, *performers of the news* rather than reporters and researchers. As a usual daily routine, only the unusually tragic or triumphant is shown—not the ordinary routines and day-to-day reality of our lives. It is true that the news show has fewer technical events. There is a good reason for this. *With fewer technical events, the news show appears realistic relative to other shows in the TV environment.* Further, it appears *super-realistic* relative to the commercial shows in this ad-vironment.

Shallow Sleep

The spectacle [media] ... ultimately expresses nothing more than its desire to sleep. The spectacle is the guardian of sleep.

(DeBord, #21)

The media guard our sleep, they proliferate and live off the will to shallowness, encouraging superficiality of awareness, triviality of being, and gossip about others as an ongoing life-occupation. The whole tone of "reporting," for example, especially on presidential elections, is often palpably adolescent and shallow. As one formula puts it, Media Power = Political Power Squared. In the political world, TV has shown us that *politicians can't be trusted*--TV can. That is, implicit in showing us this fact about politicians is the message, "We who are showing you this, the TV, *can be trusted*" (Meyrowitz 1985:268–307). Its orientation is to transform the political election into a spectacle, a celebration of amusement and a feisty, sporting, hooray-for-our-team type experience. Indeed, reporting is no longer reporting; rather, today, reporting is framing and enframing. By this we mean the media not only address the event they appear to be "reporting" on, they simultaneously teach us *how to* view the event they are reporting on: "See this election *as* a football game, see it through the same frame of reference through which you watch sports events." "See it essentially as an exciting spectacle; experience the adrenalin pumping, crowd rousing, excitement/amusement of it all."

How so are the media the guardian of sleep? Media-as-usual are thrown into stark and bold relief at those rare historical moments when an event explodes the framing. Examples of the Columbine High School mass murders or the 9/11 tragedy/murder/event come to mind. These events were experienced and reported on as events. *The whole tone, quality, texture, and composition of television changed during the coverage of those events.* The most obvious and glaring change was that *suddenly there were no more commercial message "breaks,"* no more advertisements. They just stopped. The reporters were reporting.

Everything was suddenly very, very different from television as usual, almost as if suddenly the actors, comedians, and singers in the middle of their stage performance abruptly stopped the show and just started to speak directly to the audience and to one another.

The Electronic Mind: TV and the Illusion of Knowing

> *Barbara:* Because I'm not out living in the real world, TV is my extension of that real world while I'm cooped up studying in my bedroom. I feel isolated from the rest of the world if the TV is not on.

We seem to experience TV as our eyes on the world. McLuhan says TV opens out onto an electronic global village. It would seem, rather, that it gives us the illusion of being-*there* while we never actually leave our secure and familiar living rooms. TV makes *you* the subject of everything that happens (De-Zengotita 2006:282). In a sense, on TV there are no human beings, only TV-persons, TV-heroes, TV-villains, TV-gods.

The media also confine historical reality to itself. History, as presented on television, seems to begin when television began. TV changes history in that it reflects only its own history. "The brightness surrounding the last forty years blinds us to all that preceded it ..." (McKibben 1992:64). And it limits knowledge by giving the illusion of knowledge. In the same way that the most effective way to deflect, diffuse, and terminate a social movement is to announce that it has been achieved (the feminist movement must contend with this on an almost-daily basis), the most effective way to deflect inquiry is to present it as fulfilled. TV acts in this guise as a thinking presentation device that offers up non-experience experience and not-knowing knowing. Experience becomes more and more mediated experience. "Television becomes the world for people. The world becomes television" (Mat Maxwell). The overall, cumulative effect of the media is to heighten our insensitivity to reality—especially and above all the non-human reality we are a tiny part of.

> Human beings—any one of us, and our species as a whole—are not all important, not at the center of the world. That is the one essential piece of information, the one great secret, offered by any encounter with the

woods or the mountains or the ocean or any wilderness or chunk of
nature or patch of night sky.

(McKibben 1992:228)

Rather than breaking the chains of ignorance, political domination,
and illusion in our Platonic matrix cave, something insidiously similar
yet strikingly different is going on. Being entertainment-rich, we become
knowledge-poor, acquiring the habitual mindset of a sort of impoverished
millionaire. TV is a deeply shallow experience that on some level trains
us to become more and more richly and profoundly stupid. Whereas
before we didn't know anything at all, now we "know" something that we
actually don't know. Instead of actually leaving the darkness of the cave
and going up into the sunlit reality, we merely *watch an image of ourselves
doing this—and think that is the same as doing it.*

> *Armine:*   Much to my surprise I found that the 15 minutes of watching
> nothing was MUCH MORE PAINFUL than I was anticipating. We
> truly are an entertainment oriented society. We have been trained to
> be bored if we don't have something entertaining us. We've completely
> accepted this fact and because of this we've settled for the television.

The statement "*We have been trained to be bored if we don't have
something entertaining us*" is revealing and important. Central to the
meditative, practice-oriented traditions of Buddhism is the absolute
necessity for the student to experience BOREDOM, thoroughly,
properly, and completely. Without the proper, radical, and complete
experience of boredom—opening ourselves to the experience rather
than immediately fleeing it with entertainment—the student can't
really begin to wake up to the immense and desperate preoccupation
with entertainment that is epidemic in our individual monkey-mind
and in our collective media society. The Buddhist, sociological approach
to society and self is not so much about criticizing institutions (the only
good TV is a dead TV) but about awakening from illusions. Only after
that awakening can real, effective, and genuine institutional criticism
take place and only then can social movements and social activism issue
in skillful and effective societal change.

The Truth Believed In is a Lie

There is an old slogan that goes, "The truth believed in is a lie." The outrageousness of this particular manner of expressing a "truth" is very useful. It underscores our ability to transform anything, on contact, into being anything *for our ego*. Instead of allowing truth to be, instead of letting truth be, we have a very deeply human tendency to want to own and possess it. What we mean is that the energy and relation we have to something that is true can easily degenerate and be corrupted into the energy and relation we have to *being right*. What becomes important is not the truth but the positionality of being right, being in the right and being justified and righteous.

We want to alter this ancient slogan a bit: The truth televised is a lie. Why? What sort of transformation happens such that a person, place, thing, institution or event that, if we directly experienced it, would be "true" would be what it is, yet when we experience it *as* television becomes a lie? We wouldn't say "the truth painted is a lie" nor "the truth photographed is a lie" nor "the truth radioed is a lie." Why should we here want to say "the truth televised is a lie?" We think this way of expressing it addresses and captures the essence of the view that the medium is the message. The medium is as intrinsic to the message as any content directly inscribed in or expressed by the message. When we see it on TV, "it"—whatever "it" is—is transformed from being what it is into now being a piece of TV, which is to say, in our contemporary culture, a piece of commercial entertainment.

The problem is not that TV presents us with entertaining subject matter but that TV *presents all subject matter as entertaining*. Further, all subject matter is presented as there *for us*—TV appeals to our inner-egos and we are continuously addressed, *flattered* (de Zengotita 2005), as it were, by being addressed, being broadcast to. This transcends TV and spills over into our post-TV life. TV trains us to orient toward and tune in to the entertainment quality of any experience, event, person: We look for that which is entertaining about any phenomenon rather than other qualities, like, say, depth, social significance, spiritual resonance, beauty, truth, and the like.

Howard Beale (Peter Finch) is the TV newscaster who shouts, "I'm as mad as hell and I'm not going to take it anymore!" in the film *Network*. He vividly testifies to the truth about television, namely the truth about television is that the truth does not exist in television. Today, TV doesn't imitate life, but *social life now aspires to imitate TV* (Schudson 1984:209–234). Further, as we watch television, we literally start to become greedy. Not greedy in the traditional sense in reference to money and material wealth; rather, we experience *greed for entertainment, greed for being flattered*. It becomes a 24-hour obsession. In the absence of presently occurring entertainment, we usually entertain ourselves with planning for future entertainment.

4

CONSUMERISM TV

You Are What You Want

By the advent of the 80's, Americans believed in consumption as salvation, as the only way they knew: shop 'til you drop, spend 'til the end, buy 'til you die. Buying was the new time religion, and the shopping mall its cathedral of consumption.

(Kowinski 1993:25)

Television: "All anxieties tranquilized, all boredom amused," according to the corporate cosmology of media and TV executive Arthur Jensen in the Paddy Chayefsky/Sidney Lumet 1976 film, *Network*. Everyone watches TV, but no one thinks about it. This is because watching TV precludes and short-circuits thinking about TV.

This book, being about commercial television, is by its very nature also about consuming. The culture of television that helps shape our reality, as we have discussed in the previous chapters, also creates patterns of consumption that become our reality. The curriculum of commercial television teaches us to buy to achieve fulfillment, to express our individuality and social status and, finally, to prevent economic collapse. Throughout this book, we have been looking at consuming and the mode of consumption. Whereas in most societies people work to live, in ours people work to consume. We live now in what might be called a *forced consumption culture*.

There is a rich and sustained critical tradition that has focused on media, self, and society within the context of consumerism: Vance Packard's *The Hidden Persuaders* (1954/1980); Guy Debord's *The Society of the Spectacle* (1967/1994); Marie Winn's *The Plug in Drug* (1977/2002); Jerry Mander's

Four Arguments for the Elimination of Television (1977); Ben Bagdikian *The Media Monopoly* (1983/2004); Neil Postman's *Amusing Ourselves to Death* (1985); Bill McKibben's *The Age of Missing Information* (1992); Jean Kilbourne's *Can't Buy My Love: How Advertising Changes the Way we Think and Feel (*2000); Todd Gitlin's *Media Unlimited* (2002); Mark Andrejevic's *Reality TV—The Work of Being Watched* (2004); and Thomas de Zengotita's *Mediated* (2005). All these works offer exceptionally good access to studying the culture of consumerism. Consuming is not buying what you need. It is not even buying what you want. Consumerism as an all-pervasive ideology propels the unrelenting belief that we need what we do not yet have. Consumerism is *a way of being in the world*, a fundamental frame of reference for relating to oneself, to others, and to the environment as a whole. The primary socializing force and agent behind this way of being in the world is commercial television and its embedded partner advertising. Consumerism has evolved to its present form by sharing a symbiotic relationship with television. By providing an ideal, highly enriched ad-mosphere, the social task of TV is to transform all homes into colonies of consumption.

Television: the glass tit, chewing gum for the mind, electronic alcohol, "Entertainer, painkiller, vast wasteland, companion to the lonely, white noise, thief of time...What is this thing, this *network of social relations*, called television?" (Gitlin 1986:3; emphasis ours). In the 1850s, Marx famously called religion the "opiate of the people." One hundred years later, in the 1950s, TV has perhaps replaced religion as the opiate, the Novocain, of the people.

As we have discussed, TV, non-injected, has become our culture's fundamental drug of choice: a powerful sedative to numb, tranquilize, and psychically lobotomize the alienated and dissatisfied working citizen. In terms of identity-psychology, we have almost become more consumers than workers as many people are judged—by others as well as themselves—by what they have more so than by what they do. Perhaps the seeds of this obsessive, malignant consumerism are sown in our unsatisfying, productive work lives: Because I suffer at work, therefore I will reward myself by buying. We tend to find reward through purchasing power (the paycheck and salary) rather than labor power (the artistic ability to create and make and the humanistic ability to contribute, to serve, and to make a difference).

TV amplifies our confusion regarding reality. It helps make our needs and wants ambiguous, especially through advertising. Once our needs and wants become confused and incurably ambiguous, our buying behavior becomes infinitely flexible. The primary role of most of our media today is to serve as a delivery system for advertisers. The function of the TV show is to set us up psychologically to absorb the commercial with maximum impact. The show softens, disinfects, and appropriately calibrates and focuses our minds in preparation for the injection of the advertisement. It is almost impossible these days to say *where television ends and advertising begins.*

Television and Non-Ordinary Perception

What is *the physical fixation* phenomenon at work in the practice of "watching TV?"

> In real life we perceive but a tiny part of the visual panorama around us with the fovea, the sharp-focusing part of the eye, taking in the rest of the world with our fuzzy peripheral vision. But when we watch television we take in the entire frame of an image with our sharp foveal vision. Let's say that the image on the television screen depicts a whole room or a mountain landscape; if we were there in real life, we would be able to perceive only a very small part of the room or the landscape clearly with any single glance. On television, however, we can see the entire picture sharply. Our peripheral vision is not involved in viewing the scene; indeed as the mind focuses upon the television screen and takes it all in sharply, the mind blots out the peripheral world entirely. Since in real life the periphery distracts and diffuses our attention this absence of periphery may serve to abnormally heighten our attention to the television image.
>
> (Winn 2002:26)

In terms of the physics of ordinary perception, when we watch TV we are in the presence of an anomaly, or an anomalous perceptual situation. There is an attention-binding factor present. These perceptual anomalies serve to fixate and glue our attention to the screen, and this happens on contact. There is a slight sensory confusion happening that is binding to our sensorial/cultural organization of reality. Consider the example we mentioned earlier of when you abruptly encounter a person in ordinary, everyday life whose gender is ambiguous to you. When this happens, your attention is momentarily captivated: "Is that a man or a woman?" You are momentarily stopped. The ordinary, unnoticed steam of interpretation of everyday life is suddenly interrupted and you are compelled to (1) notice and take note and (2) resolve the anomaly one way or another. You engage in fitting the person into the existing paradigm of reality (or, in moments of deep "paradigm crisis," you might stay transfixed to the "anomaly" and engage more philosophically in assumption-and-background questioning—questioning the dominant paradigm that there are and should be two and only two genders). In resolving the anomaly, you are thrust into the realm of inquiry. Your attentiveness becomes momentarily captivated in the process of investigation, and this sort of captivating investigation is on the subliminal level, as it were, as opposed to formal, full-blown conscious investigation.

Suppose we took that single moment of perplexity, confusion, and inquiry and extended it into multiple moments? Suppose we were somehow able to stretch that moment out, to repeat it again and again into a continuous process? We would have a "consciousness captivating device," a device of continuous sensory and mental confusion yet alertness. This device would enable us to *attach attention* to itself. This is at the heart of what happens when we watch television. There is a sort of short-lived hypnosis that gets recreated again and again and again, moment after moment.

Television watching both heightens attention and dulls it at the same time. There is no peripheral world of distraction and, because there is no peripheral world of distraction, our focused attention is abnormally heightened. An image in the world is quite different from the same image on television. When you see it in the world, it has a peripheral aura about it. When you see it on TV, it has no peripheral aura. Our perceptual *relation* to the image is quite distinct in our televisual experience. Because our perceptual relation to the image is heightened and exaggerated, is anomalous from our ordinary relationship to it, therefore our value relationship is also altered, heightened. If an object/person/thing is perceived in a heightened manner, it will be ascribed greater value. We're reminded of the eighteenth-century Irish philosopher Bishop Berkeley and his famous dictum: "To be is to be perceived." If we experience non-ordinary perception in the television experience, we also experience non-ordinary value and non-ordinary being.

Altering Berkeley's principle, we get "To be is to be perceived on TV." The landscape of visual perception of TV images is one that radiates and pulsates light out from inside itself. In the ordinary perceptual world, there are continuous gradations of light and shading to the objects we encounter. In the TV image, in contrast, there is a pulsating from within out onto the surface of the objects. TV objects are illuminated from within, as it were, therefore they are both *similar* to the objects in the world such that we recognize them as ordinary objects, while at the same they are *different* in that they don't quite obey the laws of perception of the ordinary material world. They are all strangely self-illuminated on the TV screen. This has a truly priceless appeal to the enterprise we call "advertising" and its obsession with the pursuit of attention.

This is all to say that what we see on the television screen is anomalously significant. What we see on TV and who we see on TV, by virtue of the non-ordinary perception that we are engaged in, take on a non-ordinary status. They are more than ordinary. They have more than ordinary being. They are celebrity objects and celebrity people. They are "stars," "brand-names," "as seen on TV."

"Watching television" then is the practice of heightened attentiveness together with the practice of confused, intoxicated, transfixed alertness. It is also the practice of structuring reality, of arranging the hierarchy of being. Socially speaking, to be on TV is to be higher on the hierarchy of attention and of value, to have fame and to be envied.

ID-TV: I Don't Want to Want, I Have to Have

With television, there is not only the immediate technology of sensory fixation and sensory attachment, there is the technology of psychological seduction and addiction. "You too can have this." "You too can be this." "This is what you want." "This is what you want to have." "This is what you want to be."…. "You want."…. "You." "Want." …. So we are in the presence of "wanting," and we are in the presence of identity, of "I" and "You." "I want." At its foundation, *commercial media shows and tells us what we want…in the mode of "I."* At its foundation, the very enterprise of commercial television assumes and believes that whatever else a television watching "I" might be, it is always also primarily a wanting being, a thing that wants. Whatever else commercial television may be showing, it is always also *telling me what I want*. Commercial television is thus at its core a *show and tell machine* (Goldsen 1977).

"I want." Let us look at this "I want," this immensely powerful and all-too-familiar experience. From the point of view of commercial media, it is of optimum value that we experience "I want" *as* "I have to have." "I want" is not experienced in and of itself, that is to say, we are not encouraged, trained, educated, or reinforced to simply *be with* our experience of wanting, of "I want." We are not encouraged to want to *experience* "wanting" or to allow "wanting" to be with us when it arises in our being. It is not sufficient to experience "I want a Barbie doll." "I want" is not really allowed to be experienced at all. There is we might almost say a strong social taboo about it. Rather, it is immediately translated into "I must have." In fact, we are afraid to experience "I want." We cannot be with wanting, that is, we cannot be with wanting *as* wanting. We must immediately—which is to say, we are deeply trained and socialized to—transform and confuse wanting with somehow purchasing, somehow consuming. We are compelled to have, we must have, we have to have. In terms of the three great categories of human life—being, having and doing—our commercial media culture collapses being and doing into having: We are what we own. If having is the same as being and buying is the same as having, then in our media culture we are in a strange way always buying being.

This whole strong tendency toward "instant gratification" is a manifestation of our acquired inability to simply be with wanting. Mostly as a result of our media training and upbringing, we experience want as unconditionally bad and gratification as unconditionally good. We don't want to want. We don't want to be with and fully experience the texture and being of "wanting." We don't want to inquire into how wanting arises in ourselves. We get almost instantly distracted from wanting into frantically having to have and thereby miss the experience and nature of wanting. In the context of our commercial media culture, wanting doesn't seek to perpetuate itself in existence: It seeks its own immediate annihilation in purchase and fulfillment. The presence of wanting as a mode of being is not entertained, experienced, nor examined. In terms of commercial media culture, we could say the same of boredom.

From this perspective, we can also begin to see why appreciation and gratitude are not qualities that are fundamentally celebrated and entertained in our commercial media. You can appreciate and be grateful for what you already have. From the fundamental design and intention of our commercial media, what you *already have* is *the enemy*—which is to say, it is that which is to be systematically discounted, de-valued, seen as old that is, no longer adequate. (Look at the hyper-degree to which planned obsolescence organizes the electronics/media/computer industry.) There will be no air time given to what you already have, nor to the various ways of appreciating what you already have. Television is not about what you already have; it's about what you don't have, or don't *yet* have. From a slightly different angle, we would also say television is not about who we already are but only who we want to be. (More on this in our mirror exercise.) This acquired training does have consequences.

Buying "Me" as Means Become Ends

Consider the all-too-familiar media voice: "Buy this item and you will be special. You will stand out from the crowd. You will express your self, your own style and your own uniqueness....And, for a limited time only, we've lowered the prices so you can *all* afford it." We are addressed as "you." As Judith Williamson (1978) analyzes in *Decoding Advertisements*, this you is a mass market "you." We are the "you" insofar as we stand in front of the ad, in front of the media vehicle. We are the "you" insofar as we participate in the entire system by "watching." There is in all this an astonishing level of mutual mass deception going on, an ongoing downy soft explosion of duplicity and confusion, of masochistic delirium and "let's pretend" submission. We are watching them, and they tell us how we can be ourselves but on a much, much better, greater, more important level. We can be a "celebrity me," totally transformed from what we are in this moment of watching, yet nevertheless safe in the consumer security of always being the familiar "me" to ourselves. We can be the same yet completely transformed. Transformed, radiant, and glamorous, yet nevertheless still us—still this familiar, comfortable...."me."

At the heart of the logic of media consumerism, the *means* to the end become the actual and real end. The means are continuously outvoting and substituting themselves for the original promised end. "'Hey You!' Buy this and your life will be transformed." "'Hey you!' If you buy this, we promise that your life will be transformed. You will become radiant, important, glamorous, envied, known, and loved by all." Of course, we go buy it, and then we *don't* experience ourselves as radiant, important, glamorous, envied, known, and loved by all. In fact, we experience a certain letdown and a certain dissatisfaction, a certain disappointment. We bought the expectation and the promise. We purchased the product (which is, in terms of re-duplication, purchasing the ad, and further in terms of meta-reduplication, purchasing and supporting the commercial media advertising system). We experience letdown and disappointment. We are not transformed, we are once again only "me." And the crucial quality of "me," of the untransformed me, is that we are witnessing others who are transformed, who are glamorous, who in *their* televisual transformation continuously remind us of our absence of transformation. The message always is not that we are not transformed but rather that we are not *yet* transformed. The unconquerable promise, the unconquerable dream, and the unconquerable possibility of future purchases are structurally absolutely necessary for this logic of consumerism, this logic of the commercial media and its counter part, the consuming self.

The more we buy, the more we are incrementally frustrated. "Every time we buy something we deepen our emotional deprivation and hence our need to buy something." (Slater 1990:103) Buying is a means to an end, which itself becomes the end. The more we buy, the less satisfied we are. The brief moment of purchase is perhaps satisfying, but the end— the transformation of our self—does not occur, not actually. We become, once again, discontented in our search for personal transformation through purchasing. Inside the cage of this hamster wheel, however, it is *impossible to become discontented with purchasing itself but only with the items purchased*. It is not the *form* of consuming that is ever questioned, just the *content* of what is consumed. Similarly, it is not the form of commercial television that is ever questioned but rather just this or that particular item or show. To question the medium itself would be to consider eliminating TV. To question purchasing itself would be to consider eliminating consumerism.

What Does Television Want? To Watch is to Want.

As one of our students was told when interviewing someone about their television watching, "I don't question television, I just watch it." Beginning to question is the doorway to all critical thinking. Realizing that we are not questioning, that we are *being non-questioning*, is the first moment of awakening. Don't question, just watch. "Just watch and just want" is perhaps the basic formula of commercial television. It is not "just want" and it is not "just watch." It is both, together: watch-and-want. The kind of watching that is promoted is the watching that wants. It is not a neutral, disinterested watching. It is not a scientific, observer-type, inquisitive watching. It is not an aesthetic appreciating watching (video art is so different from commercial television). It is more a quasi-erotic, stimulated watching: Watch, identify with, feel desire, and want. It is at its most brilliant in commercials: Watch and want. Deep inside our visual commercials is the structure: To see me is to want me. To see me is to desire me. To see me is to experience on contact the fatal attraction: "I must have you." So we have a hybrid, genetically modified watching—watching with wanting inhabiting it, from the inside as it were.

It is, we might say, the watching of the voyeur. Consider this hypothetical experience: We see our neighbors. We watch them through the window. They do not know we see them. This is a somewhat neutral version of watching. Then, unexpectedly, in the next moment, they begin to embrace and disrobe. Suddenly, our watching, the quality of our watching, and our relationship to watching change gears. Something inside the very same activity shifts, and we are watching from a wholly different psychological space. Our attachment to our watching has just amped up a number of notches. We are no longer the neutral, nonchalant, casual observer. We watch now more in the mode of wanting-to-continue-to-watch. If we have chosen to go down this route, we want to see *more*. We watch, and we want. We watch, and we want to watch, and we want to continue to watch. Our watching, as we said, is inhabited by wanting, by desiring. It is watching grounded in desire, rather than, say, watching grounded in awareness. In his analysis of *Reality TV*, Andrejevic says, "Voyeurism is an undeniable aspect of the appeal of reality TV and lends this appeal a distinct erotic charge." (Andrejevic 2004:89) It is revealing to consider that there is "a distinct erotic charge" to watching TV. Part of the appeal of this most massively common of our cultural practices is perhaps the appeal of "violating a taboo." In terms of "watching television"—below the threshold of morality, below the threshold of consciousness—we are perhaps indiscernibly, subliminally engaging in an experience of doing something we somehow feel we shouldn't be doing. Perhaps, almost imperceptibly, "feeling guilty" while watching TV is a central part of watching TV.

With television, we watch-and-want. What do we want? What do "they" want "me" to want? *What does television want?* What does our third parent want? Television wants us to want. It wants us to want what? It wants us first of all to want television. From the point of view of critical sociology, we could say that as a social institution, television serves the purpose of conditioning us to find it more and more difficult to be interested in anything *other* than television and, in this sense, having a TV makes you need a TV. From this perspective, the most important aspect of every TV show is to show the importance of TV: As McLuhan put it, the medium is the message.

TV wants us to want to stay with it, to stay tuned. As Mander says, there are always only three messages on television: Keep watching, buy something, and come back tomorrow. So the wanting is inhabited by attachment to watching and to wanting us to "buy something." Television watching is also then inhabited by buying. The relationship to buying lives inside of "watching television." We are watching and buying simultaneously. To watch is to buy. How so? The continuous, subliminal attachment to watching *is* a form of buying. What is buying? In our media culture, buying is consuming. We are conditioned to buying, and we are buying *buying* as the primary mode or relationship to have to all things.

The Internet and the Mall: "The Intermall" and the End of TV as We Know It

Having said all that, we now want to look at television in two contexts: the Internet and the mall. Consider: We are watching a show on television; we are not out at a store buying something. We are not actively consuming some commercial product. We are simply at home watching television. Let us deconstruct this socially constructed, psychologically camouflaged, highly deceptive, and ideologically permeated experience. The tiny distance that allows "watching TV" to keep its traditional character as "not actually shopping," "not actually consuming," is that we are not out at the mall, we are not "in the marketplace" scanning goods to buy. We are home in our living room, sitting on furniture, simply watching a television show. If we were suddenly transported into the marketplace, it would indeed be magical and supernatural and somewhat, of course, Internet-ish—and, needless to say, frightening and bewildering. Likewise, if we were out and about at the mall shopping and we suddenly found our self sitting "home" watching television, we would hope it was all a dream, lest we become a candidate for a mental institution. Watching TV is one thing. Shopping in the marketplace is another. These two traditionally distinct experiences are now converging, and at the design center of "watching TV" *is* buying/consuming in the market place. Consuming in the marketplace is the terminal ending of watching TV: It is that, the sake for which the television experience exists. Likewise, in terms of the dynamics of "blow back," consuming in the marketplace now deeply resembles watching television.

> Bill Gates ... envisions a world in which movies and television programs could serve not only as vehicles for product placement but also as online catalogs: "If you're watching a video of *Top Gun* and think that Tom Cruise's aviator sunglasses look really cool, you'll be able to pause the movie and learn more about the glasses or even buy them on the spot—if the film has been tagged with commercial information." The world Gates imagines is one in which actors double as catalog models and in which every item that appears in a movie—from protagonists' wardrobes to the resorts they visit—can serve as a hot-link to promote consumption....As *Survivor* producer Mark Burnett put it, the show "is as much a marketing vehicle as it is a television show. My shows create an interest, and people will look at them, but the endgame here is selling products in stores—a car, deodorant, running shoes. It's the future of television." The complete convergence of entertainment and consumption [is at hand] ...
>
> (Andrejevic 2004:43)

This "complete convergence of entertainment and consumption" that Andrejevic analyzes is at the heart of the media experience as it has been constituted for the last half-century. Media entertainment is a vehicle for marketing, a vehicle for, as one of our colleague's says, "selling soap." The endgame here is "selling products in stores." Hence, there is in all television shows a reference and connection, a direct link, to "the store." Our shows are the pathways to the stores, the shopping mall. (Our chapter on children's television shows and their relationship to the toy store addresses this.) We watch the show in the mode of buying. We track what we want. Watching and wanting are thus deeply superimposed one on the other. We consume the media, and we consume what the media stimulates us to consume. In fact, the primary definition of media today is as a space for selling and consumption. In that sense, television has always been "interactive." It has been engineered and developed and continuously improved with stimulating consumption and selling products ever in mind—not unlike the way the Internet is currently developing.

Television is visually stimulating but in a certain way. It is not primarily visually stimulating in an *aesthetic* sense but rather in a *promotional* sense. This kind of visual stimulation promotes buying, purchasing.

Survivor creator Mark Burnett's comments are richly revealing: "My shows create an interest, and people will look at them, but the endgame here is selling products in stores…" Let us break down this master formula of commercial TV. "My shows create an interest"; "people will look at them"; "the endgame here is selling products"; "in stores." To create an interest is to captivate the attention in a certain way. In what way? The way of the advertisement. Ads are designed to create an interest. They are not designed *simply* to be looked at, not even to be looked at in an informative way, they are designed to seduce us into an interest, an interest in the product on one level but more fundamentally an interest in buying, consuming. To design a "show" to be looked at with this way of looking is to design an advertisement, which is to say, a successful show *is* an advertisement. "People will look at them." People will not only look *at* them, they will look *into* them, they will "look for" in their "looking at." Hence these "show-advertisements" beckon and compel at the same time. "Look! Look at me! Look at me and want!" As we have said, this mode of looking at is always slightly tinged with the erotic and voyeuristic impulse, the erotic charge: We commonly hear "sex sells," not "information sells" or "entertainment sells." We develop and train ourselves into a certain way of seeing, a certain way of relating to this visual experience. It is a grasping, attaching, desirous sort of looking. The endgame is "buying products" and buying products "in stores." If tomorrow all stores vanished, TV would cease to exist—except perhaps TV as art form. The Internet enterprise, according to Gates's vision, is to *collapse* the "in stores" part into the "television" part. *We can purchase products while watching.* We will now fold purchasing *into* watching. *This is the sort of* "interactive" dimension—along with "multi-tasking"—that is so celebrated in much of the Internet world. "Selling products" has long been formatted into the "show" into the visual/auditory experience of watching television, and now buying products is also to be folded and formatted into the show. We will be able to "click and purchase" or "voice and purchase." To see is to shop-and-purchase. When seeing and buying become collapsed into one converged experience, commercial television as we have known it will cease to exist.

> Taken to its limit, this dedifferentiation tends toward the convergence of entertainment, advertising, and consumption envisioned by Bill Gates; every detail in every program is not just an ad but a clickable link that facilitates instant, friction-free consumption.
>
> (Andrejevic 2004:99)

There is the promise here of a complete convergence: the totalitarian convergence of entertainment and consumption. Again, Fromm's term of "unfreedom" seems to fit. Watching is buying. Buying is watching. To see is to want. We want what we see. We see in the mode of wanting it. *To consume entertainment* is thus to be *consuming the very principle of consumption*—to interiorize that which we see as exterior. To have what we behold and to become that which we behold. Reciprocally, consumption is entertainment. We entertain ourselves by consuming, and we consume to entertain ourselves.

There is, at the moment, a tiny distance between the act of consuming the televisual image and the act of shopping, of buying. There is a tiny space left yet between seeing the images on television and buying the products in the store or online. Shopping and seeing are as yet distinct practices. On this horizon, their convergence will abolish that distinction. This is a truly radical vision. As David Lazarus reported in the *L.A. Times,*

... The next big step will be shooting [TV] shows in front of green screens, allowing broadcasters to sell placement rights *after* an episode is finished and virtual sets to be digitally inserted based on advertisers' wishes. After that ... will come interactive technology to let TV viewers highlight a product on the screen and instantly receive more information. Imagine "Sex and the City" with this sort of technology. As Sara Jessica Parker cycles through designer outfits, viewers could obtain details about specific dresses or shoes, and where to buy them ... The danger, of-course, is that TV shows would become little more than virtual catalogs for advertisers, which in turn would sponsor only those programs that allowed them to display their wares.

(Lazarus 2008)

The couch potato will be not only the passive spectator consumer but the engaged discerning shopper. This "interactive freedom" is pre-structured to say the least. "Interactive" means *interactive buying*, "interactive" means shopping and choice in the realm of purchasing; hence, freedom is the *freedom to choose what to buy*. This marketing version of freedom as *freedom to choose* is the greatest ideology of our commercial media. It must be maintained so we can continue the game of advertising and marketing, so we can continue the game of selling things. If we didn't have this project of selling things, entertainment would vanish. Consuming images and television as we know it would vanish.

Television Media, The Democratic Ego, and Celebrity

Consider this statement from "webcam celebrity" Ana Voog: "It is going to be a VERY interesting day indeed when ... EVERYONE has a TV show :) I can't wait!" (Andrejevic 2005:1). As we mentioned earlier, the *desire to be on television* is one of the deep underlying structures of the *contemporary experience of television*. We want to parse McLuhan's dictum, "The medium is the message" into "Being on television is the message of television." Andrejevic's analysis in *Reality TV* addresses this dimension:

A show called *Extreme Makeover* ... rebuild[s] "real" people via plastic surgery so that they can physically close the gap between themselves

and the contrived aesthetic of celebrity they have been taught to revere
… it literally and physically manufactures celebrity-grade humans. The
power that the airbrush once exerted over the image is transposed into
the register of reality in the form of the power the scalpel exerts on flesh
… The logic is circular: the process of watching the cast members as they
are made over to look like celebrities, becomes the source of their fame
… one becomes famous by being made, both physically and symbolically,
to look famous.

(Andrejevic 2004:9–10)

Contrary to what we often hear, "reality TV" doesn't *expose* the
baseness of human beings, it celebrates it and exploits it. In that sense,
it *produces* it. In terms of social psychology and in terms of social
relationships, the fundamental experience of watching reality TV
television in our contemporary social context is voyeurism, shame, and
degradation together with glamour-and-envy. Whatever show we are
watching, we are surrounded by the haunting ghosts of our society.
Likewise, whatever societal experience we are having, we are surrounded
by the haunting ghosts of our media imprinting. The unarticulated,
unconscious message being transmitted underneath the surface of what
every "show" is showing is subliminal and subaudible. Nevertheless, it is
foundational: *You are nothing because you are not on TV.* To be on TV is
the path to being. You will go from being a "nobody" to being "famous."
Ordinary being—outside the media matrix system—is assumed to be
identical with "being nobody." Not being famous *is* being a "nobody."
Hence, the desperate and driving formula of so many of the reality
shows: It is better, of higher status, to be humiliated and degraded
publicly on television than it is to be a nobody.

If we were *just* a nobody, in some sense all would be fine, and there
would be no "problem," as it were. There would be no "issue," no space
for self-consciousness or social critique to consciously arise. However,
we as audience member are not just a nobody: We are a nobody in
the mode of adulation of famous people. It's not just that we are a
nobody but that we are a nobody in hot pursuit of being "somebody,"
which means of being "famous." To participate in this game, we must
first make our self into a nobody self, a nothing and nonentity self. We
must experience a kind of deep existential revulsion with who we are in
reference to television people. We must make our self envious of those

who possess glamour, envious of those who are media people, famous celebrities. Our fantasy project then becomes to aspire to become a celebrity star. We define the situation as we are nobody and those people on TV are somebodies. They are who we aspire to be. We do this *not* by developing, growing, and training ourselves. We can pursue this project only by being on national TV—for only then will we be the achievement of what we long for. We will be the accomplishment we long for when we first made our self into a nobody-in-the-presence-of-media-celebrity, then others who have made themselves into nobodies will envy us and want to be us. Which is to say others also will want to be-us-in-the-mode-of-being-seen-on-TV. "And who is to say otherwise in this era of the lottery of fame? Did celebrities become famous because of some inherent quality, or were they merely happened upon by the star-making industry" (Andrejevic 2004:10).

The question of whether stars become stars because of some inherent quality or because of the media machinery/industry is, from the perspective of social psychology, fairly self-evident. We never identified with the actual actor playing the character, the artist producing the performance, in the first place. What was always at work behind the projection machinery of media social psychology was identifying with the camera and the spectacle of television.

Elizabeth: Becoming an attention whore has become an acceptable job; for instance, Tila Tequila is a self-made celebrity out of this very idea. She started taking photos of herself and posting them online; the racier these photos were, the more friends she gathered. Tila became increasingly more outrageous until she was given her own television show. This reality show, A Shot At Love With Tila Tequila, was so horridly appalling that it was given a second season. Tila Tequila was given the luxurious life by spending her time becoming a whore. That sounds rather harsh, but her life's goal is to become as well known as possible at any cost. She is willing to sell herself and her love life to a television network to gain that attention; that is a textbook whore. With role models like this paraded on every network and internet outlet, it's no surprise that the vast majority of teenagers looks either like trampy starlets or self-indulgent victims of their own design. We are caught in a world of performance and it is slowly becoming an irreversible trend.

Everyone is a rock star and everyone is a celebrity…We are a generation of short-term self-oholics.

Unlike Ana Voog, we can't all have our own TV shows as then they would not be TV. The collective context of the commercial television experience is necessarily socially invidious. What we have is and can be valuable only insofar as those others don't have it and want it. If we all have this identity-defining high status symbol, it ceases to be what it is. (Give every person a Mercedes or a Rolls Royce to drive and the social status category "Mercedes" and "Rolls Royce" disappears.) In celebrity, commercial television, *our fame depends on your nobodyism and our nobodyism needs their fame.* And we both are totally dependent on the conditions of possibility for the game. The board upon which the game is played is commercial media. The source of fame and celebrity is the social relations of the commercial media industry. As C. Wright Mills noted in his 1956 classic, *The Power Elite*,

> If we took the one hundred most powerful men in America, the one hundred wealthiest, and the one hundred most celebrated away from the institutional positions they now occupy, away from their resources of men and women and money, away from the media of mass communications that are now focused upon them—then they would be powerless and poor and uncelebrated. For power is not of a man. Wealth does not center in the person of the wealthy. Celebrity is not inherent in any personality.
>
> (Macionis 1989:311)

Ourselves Diminished

To the extent that media render who we are invisible, or only show us in a negative light, they make us somehow invisible to ourselves and certainly to others around us. *The more media we watch, the less we are able to see ourselves.* Media are so central to our culture that it is very hard to know who you are or what you can be if the media give you no positive role models.

Imagine, for a moment, that the people you see on TV and in the magazines and the movies always *looked like an actual cross-section of the population*: fat people, skinny people, Black people, Asian people, Hispanic people, shabbily dressed people, pimply youths, farmers with deeply creased leathery faces, people with buck teeth and teeth missing, bald people, harassed mothers with little kids, disabled people, tired people, sick people, old people. *Would this change the way you feel about your appearance?*

Suppose we asked you to watch a few hours of TV (dramas, situation comedies, soap operas) listing the main characters and categorizing them by social class, age, appearance, and a few other variables. Then suppose we asked you to go out in public and observe ordinary people in the same way: in parks, shopping centers, laundromats, bus stations, and air terminals. You would probably find that ordinary people are not as rich, young, or beautiful as the people on TV. However, you might find that ordinary people were a whole lot more varied and interesting. Variety usually is. The real world is far richer than the sort of ideal, perfectionist realm of the media world, but media teaches us to ignore or disapprove of the richness and the diversity—to see it all merely as a degraded shortcoming from media ideals.

Perhaps the worst aspect of media's ignoring of real people is that the basic goodness and decency of ordinary people who go about their jobs, take care of their families, and contribute to their communities is totally overlooked. We believe this deeply contributes to many people's cynicism and pessimism.

If it is the case that media are "the heart of unrealism in the real world" (DeBrod 1977:13), then if the heart stops beating, the real world dies. This real world depends on the heart of unrealism. If the unrealism of the media vanished, the real world would disappear. There is a real need and a real necessity for the unrealism of the media. The real world might become intolerable without the unrealism of the media. We often hear it said, "Our economy (and hence by implication our society) would collapse without advertising." One hundred and fifty years ago, leading up to the American Civil War, it was frequently and commonly argued that although slavery was wrong, you couldn't realistically eliminate the structure of slavery as it was "necessary for the very existence of our economic system" (Fogel and Engerman 1974).

Superimposing My Face Over Clark Gable's

As we consume entertainment and entertainment in turn consumes us, we become more and more consumed by consuming and entertained by being entertained.

> Bill Gates understands that customization points in the direction not only of allowing the consumer to personalize entertainment (or news) but also of making the consumer the star: "You might watch *Gone With The Wind* with your own face and voice replacing Vivien Leigh's (or Clark Gable's). Or, see yourself walking down a runway wearing the latest Paris fashions adjusted to fit your body or the one you wish you had." The promise of customization and the promise of reality TV overlap insofar as they offer to make the viewer the star, via interactive technology... Gates, in attempting to imagine the most appealing scenario for digital customization, comes up with the promise that every where viewers look, the may find only themselves: as the stars of the shows they watch and the characters in the advertisements.
>
> (Andrejevic 2004:41)

The ideal experience that our commercial media are aspiring toward is that we can now superimpose our face literally on the screen over the face of the "stars" we are watching. (This is sort of a virtual, reverse *Celebrity Makeover*.) We are back to our original insight that the central message of our culturally formatted television experience is "you who are watching are nobody and we who you are watching are somebody." In the practice of television watching lies the aspiration to be that which you are watching while at the same time never ceasing to be yourself watching

We will be able to superimpose our face over Clark Gables face (Bill Gates' example) and insert our voice over his. We will be able to immediately buy Tom Cruise's sunglasses (again, Gates' example). Do we want to be Clark Gable, Vivien Leigh, or Tom Cruise? Not really. Rather, we want to be the character that they are portraying. We want to be *in that world*. We want to experience all this while simultaneously *never ceasing to be ourselves*. (This is somewhat like the conventional delusional practice of imagining our own death wherein we imagine our own corpse. We do all this with a good deal of skillful self-deception—

namely without noticing that we are still quite *alive* as the invisible spectator *witnessing* our dead corpse.)

We will be seen by others, by endless others. We will be seen and known and envied by others, countless others. We will be a celebrity. We will be other than who we are, other than who we are right now, right here. What does that assume about "I am?" It assumes firstly that we don't want to be "I" as "I." We want to be other than "I." This media experience drives a wedge deep into the core of our identity, of our "I." You, your "I" is nobody and nothing. This figure you are watching and identifying with is everything. It is all you could hope to be. It is all you want to be. This gives you an aspiration. This is what you want to be in the mode of not yet being it. "Not yet" is the operative term. If it were "this is who and what you want to be and aren't," that would be the end of it. It would be hopeless and depressing and final and fatal. When it ended, it would be over. But the "not yet" is the *commercial* media possibility of hope: hope that "someday" you will be. It provides the *fantasy* of possibility. We keep the fantasy alive that possibly we will one day be a star.

The commercial media experience thus is all about fantasy-toward-the-future. Not just fantasy but fantasy that could be real in the future. Not just a fantasy dream but a fantasy that is more preoccupying and lived, as it were, in the mode of entertaining it as a possibility-for-the-future, an indefinitely present fantasy project.

The Will to Believe in Progress

Scheuer, in his illuminating work on television and politics, *The Sound Bite Society*, says, "While programming has evolved in important ways, the amount and essential nature of viewing hasn't changed in a half-century" (Scheuer 1999:22). One of the primary questions our book has been probing is "What is the fundamental nature of commercial television viewing?" Another question now arises: "What is it about the essential nature of viewing, of "watching television," that has us under the spell, the deeply felt delusion that it *has* evolved, progressed, and changed radically in the last half-century?" Or, for that matter, that it has changed, progressed, and radically developed over the last 10 or even 5 years? Contrast for a moment this question regarding viewing television with "reading books." Are the books you are reading today miles ahead of the books your ancestors read? Has the amount and essential experience of reading and of reading books radically changed over the last half-century? Over the last 500 years since Gutenberg's printing press? Often, where there is no true substance, there is true hype.

Let us reframe the question and ask, "What is it about our current media culture that strongly trains and embraces us to feel and deeply believe that we are advanced over yesterday, that we are truly ahead of what things were like 10, 20 , 50 years ago." Where from—this real illusion of progress? Progress in this context is a belief, deeply held, deeply committed to, that underlies this illusion. A great principle of social psychology that we have mentioned before states, "If men define situations as real, they are real in their consequences." We today have a strong will to believe that *we are better than the past*, that *we are ahead of the past*. We emphasize this rather than that *we are the present*. Further, though it is structurally there in the background, we certainly don't dwell on the issue that we are *worse off than and behind the future*. Our media culture continuously dwells on the issue that we are progressively, linearly ahead of the past. It would seem that TV can't live without the illusion of progress. This relates to one of the great and abiding (i.e., not progressing, improving, and changing) assertions of our capitalist ideology: "You either grow or you die." This assertion we contend is mostly fear-driven. When we live from inside it, we are mostly driven by fear, by a competitive fear of failure— rather than simply growing and developing and celebrating growing and developing.

Suppose we say, "We *haven't* changed in regard to our viewing in half a century." This sounds somewhat scandalous, incredulous to our media-engorged sensibilities. From the drama and trauma of the media, we surely would have thought everything was changing and progressing … *rapidly*. We live, we are constantly told, in an age of acceleration. We are at the leading edge of the accelerating velocity of progress, improvement, and betterment.

What would it mean to say our viewing *hasn't changed*? You mean that what we experience while watching TV today is identical with what our parents and grandparents experienced when they watched TV? Suppose the media glorified the traditional, unchanging, permanent dimension of TV. "Have the same experience your ancestors did. Watch television." (We mean this point to be quite distinct from the familiar homesick, reminiscent, re-run TV: "Lets bathe ourselves in the warm flow and glow nostalgia of our common family past and our common national/ tribal past.")

What is it about our current situation that so dictates that we must, must, must define our situation as progressive, as advancing, as moving ahead? What is it that makes us fear and be repulsed at the idea that *nothing really is changing? That today is no different from yesterday?*

Entertainment Addiction

American popular culture is popular because [of]…its *commitment* to entertainment" (Gitlin 2002:206).

There is an extraordinary process of entertainment-addiction occurring in our society: One entertainment moment addicts us to the next entertainment moment and then to the next and so on. Soon we learn to entertain ourselves by looking forward to entertainment.

TV has become such a mechanical friend, such a substitute for social interaction, that our aloneness becomes acutely magnified, doubly experienced and doubly reinforced, if we are deprived of its glowing life-like presence while in the same room—as if we wouldn't still be alone if it were on. If we are alone in our room and we turn on the TV, strangely, we actually don't feel alone anymore; it's as if somehow companionship is experienced.

> *Albert:*   I just realized that whenever I'm at home I always eat (breakfast, lunch and dinner) with the television on. If I don't, I feel like a part of me is missing: my TV. Television is the only companion that never asks a thing from me. It just lets me use it for up to four hours consecutively. I feel ashamed because I could have gone out and made friends with another person, not a television.

As an advanced media culture, we seem to have achieved a new level of isolation, solipsism, and withdrawal. "It's just an object when it's turned off," hundreds of students have bemoaned in our Un-TV media exercises. When it is turned off, it more clearly reveals itself as an object, as an appliance, rather than as a friend, a companion. It is shocking after all these years to discover this. It's a little like Gass's image about an avid lifelong novel reader suddenly discovering that novels are made of words, the shock is "...as though you had discovered that your wife was made of rubber: the bliss of all those years, the pain...from sponge" (Gass 1971:27).

Mander captures well the phenomenology of the situation within which the learned practice of "watching TV" occurs:

> Television is watched in darkened rooms....it is a requirement of television viewing that the set be the brightest image in the environment or it cannot be seen well. To increase the effect, background sounds are dimmed out just as the light is. An effort is made to eliminate household noises. The point, of course, is to further the focus on the television set. Awareness of the outer environment gets in the way...Dimming out your own body is another part of the process. People choose a position for viewing that allows the maximum comfort and least motion...thinking processes also dim. Overall, while we are watching television, our bodies are in a quieter condition over a longer period of time than in any other of life's nonsleeping experiences. This is true even for the eyes—the eyes move less while watching television than in any other experience of daily life.
>
> (Mander 1977:164–165)

Almost every household's living room is arranged around the television set. As a weight room is arranged for weight training, our living rooms are arranged for TV training. The furniture is purposely arranged for the transcendent practice of "watching TV" rather than for the immanent, human practice of conversation, interaction. From this perspective, TV acts somewhat like an electronic cavity on the contemporary family and family culture: It promotes the decay of interaction and hence the decay of conversational skills. The interior design of the average American living room with its lines of attention, social organization, hierarchy, and transcendent TV is very similar to the interior design of the average American church with its transcendent altar, gestures of genuflection, and lines of homage.

Media as Worship

The TV has become our modern form of worship and ritual. The altar and ritualized ceremony of TV culture and consumption dominate our lives. It is not hard to picture the various places of media worship we have created in our homes. The family room, bedrooms, kitchens, and even the dining rooms have been organized into mini-altars that focus our attention on and interaction with our new religion. A family room that is not controlled by the media altar is almost nonexistent, not to mention how many families now eat in front of the TV. Eating or breaking bread has always been a time for social interaction. This connection is broken when we are in worship of the television while we eat. This analogy or media worship is not as far-fetched as it at first sounds. Joseph Campbell claimed that cinema had become the modern equivalent of the church in its influence on our psyche. Today's media saturated culture has made Campbell's statement more relevant than ever before.

A quick look into the average home helps illustrate this point. Not only do we situate our living areas in reverence around the TV, but TV dictates our times of social interaction. Similar to the set times to pray in religious practice (stations of the cross, praying toward Mecca five times a day), we gather at specific times to worship our new religion and take in its message communally. As we sit in awed silent reverence, the message is given. We even take our breaks at times when it is deemed suitable by the program. To an alien observer, this awed silence might even look like prayer. Even if you are alone, the act is somehow communal because thousands or millions are doing the same thing at the same time. Breaking into this ritual service is not easy. Think about trying to get something you need from someone while his or her favorite TV show is on or interrupting this individual while he or she is watching. The reaction would not be much different than interrupting a traditional worship service. Just as in traditional worship services, our responses are ritualized and predictable. This is not authentic communication but programmed behavior.

As with traditional worship services, we organize our lives around times of the service for our ritual. TV culture is a similar to Medieval church culture in this way because it is not a weekly event but a daily ritual to be performed, and it controls our entire world-view.

The community of the faithful can discuss the latest episode (sermon) with one another and feel that they are part of something bigger than themselves. Being a part of a community of believers is a very powerful part of a worship service, and the ritualized TV viewing gives a shared experience for connection to others in the same way. It is a solitary way to be social. This experience also helps eliminate some of the loneliness people feel in our society. The experience actually gives a sense of companionship and connection to others even when no actual interaction is present. It is not hard to see that our actions with the media are very similar to traditional worship services, which is why it was so easy for society to adapt to the media matrix we live in.

5

Relationship TV

I Don't Really Love You,
I Love Gordon's Gin/John Cusack

One of the Un-TV exercises we have discussed had students watch television for 15 minutes without turning it on. Through this unfamiliar, norm-breaching experience, many of them were thereby able to gain abrupt personal insight into the cultural practice of TV watching. Many became able—perhaps for the first time—to access and contemplate the subconscious background influence that TV had on their lives:

R. Walt: The time I spent staring at the blank screen was probably the hardest part of the experiment. I tried to clear my mind, but couldn't help feeling extremely uneasy. I looked at my position in relation to this thing I was staring at. I suddenly felt almost ashamed and stupid. I realized that during the most impressionable time of my life, my grade school years, I probably spent more time in this position gazing into this goddamn little box than with any other one human being. I tried to look at myself and decide what was actually me and what had become a part of me through the activity of "watching TV." To tell you the depressing truth, I couldn't discern any distinct boundaries. Perhaps it was then that I first began to get a glimpse of the immense cultural force behind this media that had instilled in me, and just about every other American, the desire to watch this thing, and thereby unknowingly adopt the values presented therein as our own.

Felicia: This 15 minute Un-TV experiment made me question the underlying motives that make us spend three or four hours a day glued to the boob tube. I found it to be a massive waste of time, yet I've done it every day for the past sixteen years of my life. Why? It seems that I have become a slave to my technology. It is as if people are obsessed with watching meaningless sitcoms and have substituted television watching for meaningful human contact. I think we have come to depend on our television sets for a kind of friendship. It makes us laugh, is mentally stimulating, and comforts us. Television never criticizes or hurts us in any way. At last people in America have found their perfect mate.

Instead of asking our students to consciously not-watch TV for 15 minutes, suppose we asked them to give up TV forever? Actually, *Life Magazine* reported a *TV Guide* poll that once did about just that:

> Would you swear off TV forever? For under one million bucks, no way. That's how nearly half of America's TV viewers feel. What's more, one-fourth of them wouldn't give it up even then. A recent TV Guide poll found that four of ten adults automatically switch on their TV when entering a room, two-thirds of the viewers eat dinner with the tube on and more than one-third use it as background noise. Also revealed: Twenty-nine percent of America goes to sleep in television's soothing glow.
>
> (Life Magazine, Dec 1992:26)

In this chapter, we explore how though television people in America have found their "perfect mate," their "perfect family," their "perfect relationship"....with television.

No Television and the Erosion of Social Bonds

In our classroom discussion, the extent to which television is eroding family bonds was once brought home to us when one student brought in an old Oprah television show—ironically enough! Several families had agreed to forego all television watching for a number of months and came back to relate their reactions to this experiment. Most of them sounded like people who had been through a tortuous, unsuccessful course of drug withdrawal. Many cheated, some couldn't go to sleep, some dreamed they were watching TV, and some wandered around lost and depressed.

However, there were also some positive stories. One family had suffered the death of a grandmother during the experiment and reported that, when they came home from the funeral, they felt at a loss without TV. The daughter said, "I wished we had TV, it would take the pain away." Instead, they sat down together and, for several hours, talked about their loss, their feelings about the grandmother, and their feelings about death. "If we hadn't been in the experiment," the daughter reported, "we would probably all have come home and gone to our individual rooms and watched television."

Families reported that they spent more time together and that children spent more time with their friends. One family went to the zoo; another got a puppy in response to TV deprivation. All of this sounded really good to us, but we had the impression that these folks didn't fully "take in" what they themselves were saying. All seemed tremendously relieved to have their TV-fix back.

Most Americans feel short of time. When asked what they miss most because they don't have time for it, the majority say that it's talking with friends and family. Putnam's *Bowling Alone: The Collapse and Revival of American Community* (2000) addresses this and related themes in great detail and depth. Yet, at the same time, we know that the average American household has the TV set on seven hours a day. Granted, as we have noted, that it isn't always being watched;, nevertheless, it is safe to assume that for three or four hours every day, people are watching it. Most of the adult watching will be done in the evenings after work, which is precisely the time when people used to talk with friends and family.

This increasing social isolation is partly due to the fact that the disintegration of the family has led to smaller and smaller living units. We as people now have fewer people to confide in. TV takes up the resultant loss of sociability. Community and neighborhood are also breaking down owing to the tremendous geographical mobility of Americans, much of it involuntary, caused by the shifting and disappearance of jobs. High crime rates keep many city dwellers, especially older ones, from going out to visit people in the evenings. Undoubtedly, TV provides these solitary-confinement prisoners with entertainment and a bond to the larger world. One must, however, question whether a screen can really replace human contact and whether we don't pay much too high a price for our mobility and for a social system that always puts economic, material production above the holistic health of the society. The lonely try to cheer themselves up by buying material goods. The supply of goods seems to justify the disruption of community. It's a vicious circle that profits the advertisers. As Wachtel puts it… "Our view of the self is that it is 'portable'; it can be carried around from place to place, fully intact, and then plugged in wherever necessary" (Wachtel 1989:120).

Mobility and physical isolation, however, don't account for all of the multidimensional transformation of replacing human contact with TV. Partly, it is the ease and convenience of TV that is so tempting. It takes a little effort to go out or invite friends or relatives over—to go to the zoo or to the meeting of a local organization—whereas with TV, it's turn on a button and slouch back in your seat. It's easier. TV asks so little of you. People are apt to give much more but also to ask more. A fatal laziness sets in. The resemblance to a drug is really not just figurative.

Television People and Real People

One of our current young American novelists, Sherman Alexie, while writing from inside the mind of a young adolescent, has his character remark, "I've never met any person who is as interesting as a good TV show" (Alexie 2007:11).

We experience our TV as our electronic companion. We have a relationship to it as surely as we have a relationship to our parents, to our friends, our lovers, our children. In Martin Buber's terms, we don't have an "I-It" relationship to TV but rather an "I-Thou" relationship (Buber 1970), and this primary, primitive relationship, this pair-bonding has come to color and permeate all our other relationships. Insofar as our relationship with this phenomenon called television becomes, in an ordinarily unnoticed way, somewhat quasi-pathological, so this "pathology-lite" grows, mutates, and infiltrates all our other relationships: our relationships with others, with our self, and with the world. It impacts, in that sense, *our relationship with relationship.* Consider that regarding our relationship with relationship commercial television functions somewhat analogously to the AIDS virus. The virus doesn't attack in any traditional way. The AIDS virus attacks not any specific site in the body but rather the body's ability to detect and defend itself against alien attacks. Most viruses attack some dimension of the body and, in response, the body's immune system kicks in at the first recognition of these alien invaders and so begins the various fights to maintain the integrity and the health of the body. If the immune system is successful—both in itself and in marshalling the forces of the body—the body returns to health; if the immune system is unsuccessful, the body expires. AIDS, however, *attacks the immune system itself.* There is no immune system to protect the immune system. In attacking and compromising the immune system itself, AIDS harms and kills by leaving the body completely vulnerable to any opportunistic disease that comes along. Commercial television, we are arguing, has similarities. It impacts our "relationship system" the way AIDS impacts our immune system. In this chapter, we explore how our relationship with television affects our relationship with relationship.

People today feel deeply connected to people they don't know, to "media people." We contend that as we connect more and more to the unreal, or quasi-real media people whom we don't know, we disconnect more and more from the real people that we actually do know, interact, and live with. "For surely the hours that children spend in a one-way relationship with television people, in involvement that allows for no communication or interaction, must have some effect on their relationships with real-life people" (Winn 2002:158). In the television world, and now more and more in the Internet world, many of us feel we are somehow experiencing an in-depth meaningful relationship without ever actually meeting the other person. It is a connection, but it is mediated connection, not an interactional relationship. It is rather a quasi-solipsistic, techno-relationship—relationship-lite, if you will, however intense it may actually feel.

Consider what one student realized when given the assignment to "consciously reflect upon their most significant childhood relationship with a television character" (more on this assignment in the Saturday Morning Ghetto chapter):

Caroline Lucas: Ariel is more than just a red-headed, finned, purple-shelled princess of the ocean. She is my ultimate idol and has been since the age of two years old. I can distinctly remember the day that I got Disney's The Little Mermaid on tape as a birthday present from Grandmamma. I must have watched that video at least a thousand times over the next sixteen years of my life….Ariel and the story of her journey of being a mermaid to becoming human has become a reoccurring theme throughout my childhood…My love for Ariel and her plight as a mermaid princess may have faded as I grew out of my childhood, but it resurfaced this first year at college…when I walked into Disneyland ten years later all of these childhood memories came flooding back to me. When I passed by Ariel's Grotto and she was sitting there taking pictures with all the little kids, I honestly became a little too excited for someone who is almost twenty years old. At least I had the self-discipline to not jump in line for a picture…It just really surprised me how much I still adored this imaginary figure, even ten years later. My idolization, admiration, and even love for this cartoon sketch were startling and a little frightening.

Even as I write this paper, I sit listening to the entire soundtrack from the movie … Just by listening to the music I can picture every scene in my mind, recite lines from the film and know every word to every song by heart. The film is ingrained in my mind not just because I enjoyed the story, but because I wanted to be Ariel, a beautiful mermaid princess with a fairytale romance and a happy ending. Through the powerful imagination of my youth, I was able to live in her world through watching the movie, creating scenes with the dolls and dressing up in her attire. She not only provided an escape, but an ideal of how life and romance should be. The sad thing I am now realizing is that all this time and energy resulted from not even a real person, but a fabricated media character created by a giant, evil corporation. What's even sadder is that this realization still isn't going to stop me from buying The Little Mermaid when it is released on DVD from the Disney Vault. At least I will admit this painful fact.

Again and again, we found with our students a real intensity of attachment and imaginary involvement with the media figures of their childhood. We also found this same phenomenon when assigning our students to go out and interview pre-schoolers about their experience of "television-people:"

Alex: Kylie is three and a half years old and …is very articulate for her age … . I asked what her favorite TV show was. Kylie was quick to answer, as if she had been expecting it—Dora the Explorer. I asked her why and she replied, "Because Dora is … smart and … . I like her. She goes places, and I go too…and I have her stuff." The tone in her voice changed as she was answering this question, as if she were considering Dora, outside of the TV show, as a real person. Probing further, I asked whether she and Dora were friends. "Um, yeah," she replied. I thought back to the types of shows I used to watch and wondered whether I had ever considered myself to be "friends" with anyone on those shows. I asked her whether she and Dora went places together. "Yes!" she chirped emphatically. "Has she been over to play at your house?" I asked. "No," Kylie said, very matter-of-factly. "And why not?" I inquired. I'm assuming I caught her off guard as she made a little whizzing sound and did not reply. I asked again, rephrasing just in case, "Kylie, how come you don't invite Dora over to play at your house?" After a couple seconds, she replied, "She's on TV." At this point I got very excited and was eager to probe Kylie's "relationship" with Dora after such a statement, but I became worried that I might upset or confuse Kylie by pointing out this impossible situation. "Kylie," I began, "do you and Dora talk to each other?" "Yes," she replied. "When does she talk to you?" "On the TV … she talks to me." She still had the same excited, warm tone in her voice, as if she were talking about someone she truly liked or cared for … ."Does Dora talk to your mommy and dad too?" "Yeah." "Where?" No response. I waited a couple of seconds before rephrasing, "Kylie, does Dora talk to your mom and dad?" "I don't know … yeah … no." I could tell she was done playing with me. I thanked her for talking to me…After talking with Melissa, Kylie's mom, for a few minutes, I learned that Kylie's room is decked out in wall-to-wall Dora stuff, from her Dora backpack to her Dora comforter … . I don't know for a fact whether or not Kylie thinks Dora is real. Although she spoke about Dora as if she were in fact, real, the confusion I caused her with some of the questions leads me to believe that she does not think, at least without doubt, that Dora is real. This does not mean, however, that she does not think that she has a real relationship with Dora. What is necessary to have a relationship? You must see the person, or at least imagine the person physically, Kylie sees Dora everyday. You must be able to interact with the person; Kylie has real experiences with Dora through "interaction" with the show. Kylie learns as Dora "learns" on the show. They go through events and experience adversity in real time—together—because of the way the show was designed. I think it is entirely possible that Kylie and Dora have a relation ship because of this fact alone. So then Kylie does not have a relationship with TV, but rather a relationship with someone very real—because she, Dora, was created to be as real as possible.

Media Imprinting: I Don't Love You, I Love John Cusack

> What a child learns from a parent is how to have a relationship.
>
> (Carnes 2001:59)

We want to develop this theme of our relationship to relationship now by looking at a disturbing statement that Marie Winn made originally in 1977 in the very first edition of her classic work on the impact of television on children, *The Plug-in Drug, Television, Children and the Family*. This work was revised and updated in 2002 in a 25th anniversary edition as *The Plug-In Drug, Television, Computers and Family Life*. (We will be repeating her statement a number of times.) Winn's statement addresses the "imprinting" phenomenon made by television on very young children. The phenomenon of imprinting was richly articulated by the renowned twentieth-century ethologist Conrad Lorenz. He studied how graylag geese that just hatched out of incubated eggs would imprint or "attach" to the first figure that they came across within about 36 hours of their birth. They took Lorenz himself—actually his boots—*as their parent* and followed and imitated him *for the rest of their lives* (Lorenz 1982). In Winn's study, this peculiar form of electronic media imprinting haunts these children—who are, of-course, all of us—their entire lives. After Winn's statement, we want to look at a long description Chuck Klosterman wrote in his self-reflective 2004 work, *Sex, Drugs and Coco Puffs*, regarding the media and the contemporary cultural predicament of "falling in love." We will see Klosterman as examining the transformation love undergoes when it becomes love in the age of television.

First Winn:

> To a certain extent children's early television experiences will serve to dehumanize, to mechanize, to make less *real* the realities and relationships they encounter in life. For them, real events will always carry subtle echoes of the television world (2002:13).

Now Klosterman:

> I once loved a girl who almost loved me, but not as much as she loved John Cusack. Under certain circumstances, this would have been fine; Cusack is relatively good-looking, he seems like a pretty cool guy ... and he undoubtedly has millions of bones in the bank. If Cusack and I were competing for the same woman, I could easily accept losing. However, I don't really feel like John and I were competing for the girl I'm referring to, inasmuch as *her relationship to Cusack was confined to watching him as a two-dimensional projection*, pretending to be characters who don't actually exist ... . It appears that countless women born between 1965 and 1978 are in love with John Cusack ... . But here's what none of these...women seem to realize: They don't love John Cusack. They love Lloyd Dobler. When they see Mr. Cusack, they are still seeing the optimistic, charmingly loquacious teenager he played in *Say Anything*... We all convince ourselves of things like this ... . *This is why I will never be completely satisfied by a woman, and this is why the kind of woman I tend to find attractive will never be satisfied by me.* We will both measure our relationship against the prospect of fake love. Fake love is a very powerful thing ... Pundits are always blaming TV for making people stupid, movies for desensitizing the world to violence, and rock music for making kids take drugs and kill themselves. These things should be the least of our worries. *The main problem with mass media is that it makes it impossible to fall in love with any acumen of normalcy* (2003:2–4 emphasis added).

A whole series of possibly disturbing questions comes to mind: Does television, or rather, does our relationship with television, somehow make us unable to have a true, real relationship with another human being? Does our relationship with television actually do damage to our relationship with real people? Does our relationship with television somehow incapacitate, or somehow render ineffective, our relationship with people? Does our relationship with electronic media technology negatively impact our relationship with living people? How does our media relationship with the fantasy characters on television affect our relationships with the real people in our life. How does our *identification* with media characters (we want to be like X) affect our identification with real people? How does our *desire* for media characters (we want X) affect our desire for real people? Are we condemned to compare our happiness or our ideas of love with what is portrayed in the media? Does a "healthy" relationship with television promote our having healthy relationships with the real people in our life?

Relationship

How does our relationship with television affect our relationship with relationship? Assume, for a moment, that at the heart of our self, at the very core of who and what we are, is not "self" but rather "relationship," not a "thing" but a "happening," not "matter" but "space." This assumption echoes the lines of Kierkegaard's famous opening in *The Sickness Unto Death,*

> Man is spirit. But what is spirit? Spirit is the self. But what is the self? The self is a relation which relates itself to its own self, or it is that in the relation which accounts for it that the relation relates itself to its own self; the self is not the relation but consists in the fact that the relation relates itself to its own self.
>
> (Kierkegaard 1941:146)

Let us also here take seriously, for a moment, Marie Winn's view that at the social core of our existing television experience is some hitherto-never-before-existing drug: *The Plug In Drug.* What happens if we locate our reflections on television, self, and relationship more deeply inside the context of drug addiction and recovery? What is *the addicts relationship to relationship?* An addict is someone who is addicted to X (a substance, a behavior, an experience). If, as an addict, our *primary* relationship is to a substance, we are somehow *no longer grounded in the human to human relationship world.* That core existential fact will saturate the tap-root of our relationship to people. We will, over time, begin to reduplicate and replicate our relationship with our substance inside of our relationship with people. There is an astonishingly powerful statement in the "Big Book" of Alcoholics Anonymous (2002) to the effect that "We believe that at the heart of our disease is our inability to form a genuine relationship with another human being." For the addicted person, the heart of their world and their reality is their relationship with their substance. Patrick Carnes notes in his *Out of the Shadows, Understanding Sexual Addiction,*

A common definition of alcoholism or drug dependency is that a person has a pathological relationship with a mood-altering chemical ... To feel "normal" for the alcoholic is also to feel isolated and lonely, since the primary relationship he depends upon to feel adequate is with a chemical, *not other people.*

(Carnes 2001:14; emphasis added)

For addicted persons, their relationship with the fundamental phenomenon of relationship itself is deeply distorted, deeply dysfunctionalized into relationship with a substance rather than a person, a relationship with a "thing," as it were, rather than with a person. Let us translate this issue into the I-Thou relationship language and categories of the philosopher Martin Buber. I-Thou is a human relationship between two conscious and aware people who acknowledge their mutual humanity. I-Thou means I-You. I recognize you as another I, an other I. As an addict, the foundation of our life and of our social, interactional world, eventually comes to rest on an abnormal "I-It" relationship rather than a normal "I-Thou" relationship. Our fundamental orientation of I-It will, like a secret parasite, inhabit all of our I-Thou relationships. If at the foundation of "my relationship to you" is my groundedness and my deep training in my relationship to "It," my substance, my drug, I am not really in a human relationship, a real human relationship, with you. However subliminal, hidden, and disguised it may be, I, as an addict, am in an instrumental relationship with you, with "Thou." Behind "you" lies "it." Behind my surface experience of you lies my deep experience with it. Again, let us listen to what Winn is saying,

To a certain extent children's early television experiences will serve to dehumanize, to mechanize, to make less *real* the realities and relationships they encounter in life. For them, real events will always carry subtle echoes of the television world.

(Winn 2002: 13)

After almost 80 years of 12-step recovery work—which was begun by Alcoholics Anonymous in 1935—it has become abundantly clear that those people who are not themselves addicts but who know, love, and are in intimate relationship with addicts—the Alanon movement— have a very, very difficult challenge to face. To put it in the direst terms, their addict loved one is incapable of having a real human relationship with them. Their addicts' attempts at having a real, human, interactional, I-Thou, partnership relationship with them will continuously be "outvoted," as it were, by the addicts' fundamental relationship to their substance, an addictive "I-It" relationship. As addicts, they relate to you in the mode of getting high off of you, as they relate to their drug. It's not *you* they relate with but the *effect* you produce on and in them; hence the central issue of "selfishness" and "narcissism" are seen at the heart of the psychology of addiction and of recovery from addiction.

If an individual is in an addictive relationship to television and that addictive relationship becomes foundational for their experience of life, "television fundamentalism"—four hours a day of focused watching, the greatest "occupation" other than work and sleep; seven ours a day the set is "on" in the background—then when they relate to you, certain things will be present. Rather like the character Dianna Christianson in the film *Network* that we addressed in Chapter 1, *they will relate to you somehow, however subtle it may be, as* another *TV experience.* They will somehow, in a mostly unconscious way, be relating to you as another TV character, another TV show, another TV experience. They will have, in deep unawareness, certain expectations that they project onto you, or more precisely, "You." We put quotes around "you" here because active TV addiction makes all you's into "you's." People are now "people," not quite real in and of themselves. "You" are to entertain them. "You" are the entertainer and the entertainment. "You" are the medium of entertainment. "You" are here to produce an effect on them or to generate a high in them. And "you" can be switched to another "you" at any moment.

I Don't Love You, I Love Gordon's Gin

The topic of "relationships" is frequently discussed in 12-step recovery meetings around the world. In the context of working with their addictions, the question is often posed by people who are in recovery, "How has my drinking affected others?" Or, more broadly, "How has my addiction to X caused damage to others?" As a general example of addiction, let's focus on alcoholism. Alcoholism is defined as a family disease and malady. Toward the end of one AA meeting we attended, a prosperous looking gentleman struggling with his recent sobriety shared about how whenever the situation arose that he had some time alone away from the other members of his immediate family, he viewed that situation as "his time to drink." He went on to say that Tuesday nights his wife goes out to teach law and doesn't come home until 11 PM. He looks after his young daughter, and he tries to get her in bed early so that he can drink. Then he really hit upon something very raw regarding the relationship psychology of addiction. He confessed, *"Whenever I would say to my daughter, 'I love you,' my immediate next thought was 'No I don't. I love Gordon's Gin.' Whenever I said to my wife, 'I love you,' my internal dialogue would say, 'No I don't. I love gin. I love drinking.'"* We saw in his sharing the truth of that statement in the "Big Book" of Alcoholics Anonymous mentioned earlier that "at the root of our disease is our inability to form a true relationship with another human being." For the addicted person, at the root of their dis-ease is *dis-ease in relationship*; at the root of their malady is their sick relationship to relationship itself, above all to the primal relationship called "love."

Let us now extend and apply this perspective to our relationship to television. *How does our relationship to television impact our relationship to love, to our love relationships? In Sex, Drugs and Coco Puffs*, when Klosterman's beloved says to him "I love you," his very next thought is "No you don't. You love John Cusack." To the degree that we cultivate and grow ourselves into an "addictive" relationship with the media, with television, a "dis-eased" relationship, we become less and less capable of having a *real* love relationship with another human being, which is to say we become incapable of having a love relationship with a *real* human being. In the contemporary cave of the media matrix, we've reduced ourselves into loving shadows on the cave wall. *"This is why I will never be completely satisfied by a woman, and this is why the kind of woman I tend to find attractive will never be satisfied by me.* We will both measure our relationship against the prospect of fake love. Fake love is a very powerful thing ..." (Klosterman 2003:4).

Let us reflect further on Klosterman's insights. "Yes, yes," we may say to ourselves, "I know that 'I love you.'" or "Yes, yes, I know that 'You love me.'" Nevertheless, *something is off.* Something is not really right. It's not whole, complete, and true. You are not *free* to love—even though you may protest that you are. Yes, you would like to love me, but

I know that you love John Cusack more. Your ability to love me as one human being to another has been fatally compromised. Compromised by what? Compromised by your relationship to the media, to television. You will be loving me (the real person me) *within the context* of your media relationship to John Cusack and to your relationship to the world that John Cusack inhabits and makes visible, your relationship to media love, to "fake love." You now love the world of love as you have been imprinted, as you have come to know it in the media, in television. *That* is true love. That is what you truly love. That is who you truly love.

When your true love, or your first love, is a "what" rather than a "who" (An I-It rather than I-Thou), love itself is fatally altered, mortally wounded, deeply dysfunctionalized and disordered. It is a deadening love rather than an enlivening love, a love of expectations rather than of openness, a love guided by "expectance" rather than acceptance. It is a love, strangely enough, grounded on isolation—the isolation formed of deep passivity and spectatorship—rather than a love of communication and contact. In this love world, I can only be alongside of you, rather than *with* you.

Let's say that we are with our wife, our beloved, who is alcoholic, and she takes a drink. Suddenly, we are no longer with her in the same way. She gets "taken away" from us by her real "love"—alcohol. Something instantaneously transforms in her, and she is no longer who she is. There's somewhat of a Jekyll and Hyde transformation. She is no longer her self. She is now Other.

If our primary love imprint is derived from the media, if our root human capacity to love is somehow diverted and dysfunctioned onto an "animated object," onto a "life-like machine," onto a virtual, parallel celebrity universe, then when we say "I love you" to another person, when we say I love you to our wife, to our daughter, to our father, we know somewhere in the depths of our psyche that we are lying: I love you but I love gin more. I love you but I love John Cusack more. Whomsoever I love, I don't love, I can't love, because I love my addictive substance more. We are imprisoned inside our primal addictive love relationship. Love, our love relationships, the root avenue and the fundamental open pathway of growth and development hereby become transformed into an endlessly recreated, hamster wheel prison of dysfunctional, neurotic love. Again, even at the risk of over-repeating ourselves, let us revisit Marie Winn's statement about children and television.

> To a certain extent children's early television experiences will serve to dehumanize, to mechanize, to make less *real* the realities and relationships they encounter in life. For them, real events will always carry subtle echoes of the television world.
>
> (Winn 2002: 13)

Romantic Love

In the contemporary arena of "romantic love," the machinery of projection is indeed deep and intractable. Under earlier, pre-electronic circumstances the whole human phenomenon of "falling in love" was already soaked through and through with the machinery of projection, and "love-at-first sight": You somehow awaken in me a dormant seed of yearning, of "falling," and I stop seeing you and start "projecting" you, projecting upon you. This psychological projection is deep, primitive, and powerful. Add onto this root psychological projection the phenomenon of visual electronic projection and the problem becomes intensified. The figure on the screen—or the cave wall—is literally a projection. We identify with a projection. We identify most in the mode of wanting to be (identification) or in the mode of wanting to have (desire). *Habitually* identifying *with a projection again and again makes us in turn more of a projection our self. Wanting to* have *a projection also makes us more of a projection our self.* In the media matrix cave of shadows, we become more of a shadow ourselves. So now our projecting onto others in the arena of "romantic love"—an arena already grounded upon psychological projection—becomes a double projection.

This culture-wide, socially reinforced media addiction, this all-pervasive network of expectations keeps us deeply imprisoned in the ever present media preoccupation of "looking for the right person"—even after we've found the right person. The problem with being imprisoned inside of "looking for the right person" is that it is a media, consumerist driven delusion—with planned obsolescence folded into it. On a fundamental level, you can't really *find* the right person. In the non-media, *human* world of actual interaction, actual love, and actual relationship, you can't *find* the right person, you can only *be* the right person.

Family Dysfunctional

> I must begin by making a distinction between a technology and a medium. We might say that a technology is to a medium as the brain is to the mind. Like the brain, a technology is a physical apparatus. Like the mind, a medium is a use to which a physical apparatus is put. A technology becomes a medium as it employs a particular symbolic code, as it finds its place in a particular social setting, as it insinuates itself into economic and political contexts. A technology, in other words, is merely a machine. A medium is the social and intellectual environment a machine creates.
>
> (Postman 1985:84)

If we live in a dysfunctional family, we become dysfunctional. We *learn* to be dysfunctional. It is a quality of being that we help grow through our acquired interactional patterns. It is not a quality of being that we more or less mechanically inherit from the outside, as it were—like our eye color. It is a quality of being that we actively participate in and relate to grow and develop; hence we are involved with participation, with learning, and with practice. Consider, for a moment, that *living with a television* in the household *is living with a dysfunctional family*. It is in the relationship to television that the dysfunctionality develops, rather than in the TV technology itself, as an external, indifferent object.

When we think about love today, we automatically think media, which is to say we think in the grammar, lexicon, and rhetoric of commercial media. In our media culture, we have this fantasy story angle of approach to love relationships, rather than a real, manual, hands-on approach to love relationships and to working through and living in love relationships. Rather than a family-grounded schooling-and-curriculum in relationship realities, we have a media-grounded schooling-and-curriculum of relationship delusions. *In our media-wired, cabled households, every family member is frequently in a TV relationship first and a family relationship second.* If we are first co-spectators and only second interactants, we don't really learn about our love relationships from our family interactions and interrelationships but rather from our media spectatorship envelopment and enmeshment.

Love

We learn from the TV, and we learn from others how to relate to the TV. We learn from the relationship that others have to TV to develop our own relationship to TV. Relationship is the key element: the relationship of spectating, the relationship of emulating the electronically projected, the relationship of relating to TV as real and hence also of relating to the real as TV—"Reality TV" and "TV Reality." If our relationship to TV and our relationship to reality are intermixed, we have reality TV and TV reality. We have neither TV nor reality but now this peculiar hybrid. "The main problem of the mass media is that it makes it impossible to fall in love with any acumen of normalcy" (Klosterman). Why? Because media *de-normalizes reality*. The media de-normalizes the normal. Through its relentless pursuit of glamour and excitement, it transforms the normal into "normal," into that which is devalued (more on this in our looking glass self chapter). Whatever *is*, is unsatisfactory. It is unsatisfactory *because it is*. Our relationship to reality is dysfunctionalized because reality is now experienced as unsatisfactory. "What's so great about reality?" a techie friend of de Zengotita once said to him (deZengotita 2005:203). Existence in the world is unsatisfactory. It is not glamorous. Media is glamorous, media is interesting, media is true being--TV is true being. TV dysfunctionality is characterized by having a weak relationship to the satisfactory level of being—that is, of what is and of what is actually occurring in the present moment.

We experience the real world in the context of the television world, and the real world is found wanting. It is dissatisfactory, rather than satisfactory. In this dialectical whirlpool, the alchemy of TV produces a sort of global dissatisfaction with reality. In this sense, TV generates a micro-millimeter, transparent film layer that subtly insulates and distances us from immediate contact with reality, and especially from contact with the self-existing, satisfactory nature of reality. We are just ever so "slightly off" *continuously*. Our internal "voice" has been hijacked by television and television portrayals such that whatever is actually going on with reality, or with the real person we are in a love relationship with, is, in and of itself, "off," unsatisfying. "This is why I will never be completely satisfied by a woman, and this is why the kind of woman I tend to find attractive will never be satisfied by me" (Klosterman). On its own, it is unsatisfying, which is to say it is unsatisfying in reference to our TV-conditioned fantasy generator continuously humming in the background. This humming is projecting, expecting, measuring, comparing, and *pre-experiencing* the actuality of what is occurring and forever finding it ... unsatisfying.

Love and the Media

Our ideas of love have been so distorted by the media that it has become almost ridiculous. The idea of romantic love has been manipulated and bastardized to the point at which it effects the relationships we are a part of. We have been bombarded since childhood with media propagated love ideas: that we can find the "one" person out there for us, that we will one day experience love at first sight or that love conquers all. These ideas are so engrained in our minds that it doesn't register to most people that love and relationships take time and work to be successful and that what we see in the media isn't real relationships but myth. Many couples actually break up because they "just don't feel the fireworks anymore" or this person wasn't the "one" as they continue in vain to search for their Prince or Princess Charming. Because their love life didn't resemble the media paradigm, it must not be real love, or this must not be the "one."

This love myth phenomenon has been taken to a new extreme in reality TV. Millions of people tune in each week to see whether the Bachelor or Bachelorette will find true love or maybe Joe Millionaire, or Joe Schmo. The idea that love can be a game show or something that can be found in a few weeks by dating 30 different people in a highly controlled and contrived setting is frightening. We believe it also indicates how deeply this myth of love that the media has fed us our entire life is now a part of society's fabric. People watch these shows and the contestants with such fervor and passion, even more than if they were their own family or friends, as they date and find "love" in front of the world.

In today's political landscape wherein the debate about what should constitute marriage can dominate a political campaign as much as world events or the economy, it is amazing that these shows even exist. The absurd view that meaningful "true love" is going to be found in a manufactured TV event is more disturbing and degrading to the institution of marriage than almost anything conceivable, and it is surprising that they haven't become political fodder instead of media institutions. This again can be used to illustrate the power of this distortion in our consciousness. These shows are just modern adaptations of the way we have been fed the love myth our whole life. Cinderella and Sleeping Beauty have been turned into speed dating for Prince Charming for an attention-deficit society. The Bachelor/Bachelorette even goes to the extreme and, in the end, a marriage proposal ring ceremony takes place. Yet, almost all of these love-struck couples don't even make it to the final taping together because they find out without the TV crew and fantasy-dating situation that they don't really have much together. Love is a gift and one of life's greatest experiences, but the distortions that the media push on society makes a mockery of what love is. You have to wonder what effect our long-term exposure to these ideas does to our understanding of love and our experience of healthy relationships.

TV Character Relationships

Through a variety of exercises, we provoked our students to begin to critically, consciously reflect on the TV characters that they actually formed relationships with. In this critical and therapeutic process much was revealed:

Emily: When I set out to write about my relationship with Bridget Jones, I encountered a problem. It's not so much that I have a relationship with Bridget Jones, it's that I am Bridget Jones. Well, of course, I know that I'm not actually Bridget Jones (as she is fictional), but as I jokingly say to my friends, we are so similar that I may as well be. So writing about my relationship with Bridget Jones would be like writing about my relationship with myself, and how can I do that? That's when it hit me: is this not the point? I've identified so strongly with this character that I've embraced her as a facet of myself, an extension of my personality. What does this say about my emotional availability to the media?

Kathryn: My relationship with Clarissa (Mellissa Joan-Hart) began at the ripe young age of seven. Although I cannot remember my first contact with her, I remember the budding of our relationship well. In the first few weeks after seeing her, Clarissa was an icon for me. She had the coolest clothes and I soon began wanting to follow a similar style. She listened to Pearl Jam and attended their concerts , and even though I didn't know who Pearl Jam was and had certainly never heard of them, I instantly like them. I still remember the first time I actually heard a Pearl Jam song; it was almost five years after the end of Clarissa, and yet I immediately liked the song because I knew it used to be Clarissa's favorite band. Clarissa's younger brother, Ferguson, used to really bug me too. I always used to get so frustrated with him, saying, "Fergie was SO annoying today! I can't believe how much of a brat he is!" That's when I realized that Clarissa was more than just an icon; she was a friend. It is as if Clarissa had become my older sister and a knowledgeable influence...

Looking back on our relationship, I realize just how much influence Clarissa had on my beliefs and personality ... . It is scary to think that my lifestyle choices could have been influenced by a TV character, or worse, a TV friend. It is especially unnerving for me as someone who longs to be an individual and not consumed with the flow of the crowd...

It is ironic that Clarissa, as a TV personality, had such a rebellious attitude. The entire essence of TV is conformity: without high ratings, shows don't survive. So how many other children were affected by Clarissa, and how many more are still influenced by her even though she has disappeared from the magic box? I know for a fact that when I talk about Clarissa today, most of my friends remember her ... . The most amazing thing is that even though all of my real friends didn't watch Clarissa with me those years ago, they had many of the same emotions and reactions toward her. This concept is incredible. How could we all have had the same relationship with someone when we didn't have a relationship with each other

Alex: For much of my early adulthood, one character in the media really stands out as having the largest impact on my life. Dwayne "The Rock" Johnson, as seen nearly every week on the WWE, is someone who I believe I have had a "relationship" with for as long as I have watched wrestling and beyond. Although it has been about three years since I've stopped watching wrestling (I'm 20), I feel my relationship with The

Rock is still as fresh and solid in my mind as some of the relationships I have had with teachers, mentors, and several other "real world" role models. The Rock was more than just a role model to me—he was a way of life. That is not to say I worshipped him as a person, but rather the things he accomplished both on stage (and in the ring, if you will), and off ... . I respected The Rock as both a wrestler and entertainer, and now I respect the man as an actor. But our relationship evolved over time. At first, I approached the Rock as a fan. I enjoyed watching him wrestle and trash talk the other wrestlers, but he was not someone I looked up to initially. It wasn't until my mood became affected by how well he had performed the night before or if he had been cheated out of a win that I started to notice myself being sucked into the realm of pro-wrestling. I remember jumping off my couch and being totally crushed if he didn't win. What's more, I remember attributing a two-month period of depression in my 8th grade year to The Rock turning "heel" (the wrestling term for bad-guy). Today I often attribute The Rock as being the sole influence for my charismatic acting and public speaking abilities. Although I no longer watch wrestling and The Rock no longer wrestles, I believe our relationship is still as valid as it was four years ago.

My Ego Space

Can hundreds of millions of people be wrong? The amazing rise of the *Myspace* and *Facebook* phenomena is almost hard to believe. In a few short years, these social networking sites have become some of the most popular sites in English and even in the world. *Myspace* and *Facebook* are homes to various music, film, book, blogs, videos, and school information avenues but are known primarily for their user profiles as a way of communicating with "friends." In a few years, an idea has overwhelmed the expectations of everyone (*Myspace* was bought by News Corp and Rupert Murdock for $580 million, and Google has announced it will pay $900 million to be able to advertise and search for the site) and, for many of the young, it has transformed the way people talk to each other. *Myspace* and *Facebook* have become almost necessities for social survival in many circles.

As most of you reading this already know, each registered user profile has two customary "blurbs" associated with it: "About Me" and "Who

I'd Like to Meet." Here the user can create a page about their interests, including music, TV, movies, books, hobbies, and the like and upload images or videos of themselves to attach to the profile. A count of the user's friends is also included as is a "Top Friends" area, which of course has been known to cause fights among the "friends" for the order they are in. Below this area is also a comment section wherein friends can leave comments about the user for all members to read. It is up to the user to either leave these for public display or to edit out their personal business. Some have turned this site into a business and parlayed their huge number of "friends" into lucrative commercial efforts. A certain Christina Dolce, the networking "friend" queen, has capitalized on her million "friends" to sign deals with companies such as Axe body spray and Zippo lighters, not to mention her $5,000 personal appearance fees.

Many people involved in *Myspace* and *Facebook* claim that it actually keeps their friendships closer. They communicate more often and that it is a beneficial way to maintain friendships in our busy lives. Ironically, a 2006 study in the *American Sociological Review* (McPherson, Smith-Lovin, and Brashears 2006) found that American's now claim to have a third fewer intimate friends and confidants than 20 years ago. Twenty years ago, individuals claimed to have three close friends to share with, and that has now dropped to two. Further, 25 percent of the respondents claim to have no one at all. That is a very significant change; our social networking safety net seems to be shrinking even though *Myspace* and *Facebook* and other cyber social networking sites would lead you to believe otherwise. It seems cyber or cell phone contact with friends is a hollow replacement for face-to-face human interaction. This information points to some important questions. Even though communication is happening, what type of interaction is it? Is this interaction actually helping to build friendships? Does the non-verbal nature of the communication distort or change the relationship? Are users communicating only with their already established "friends," or are they now involved with many people they have never met except in cyber space? How do these interactions with cyber friends affect relationships with close friends whom you are in contact with outside cyber space? How can we know whom we are meeting when all we know about the person comes from a page full of things they chose to put on their space? How much of the information that is put on the sites is really only what we want people to see about us? Are the people who find our sites attracted only to what we say we are like?

Freud believed our ego worked on a reality principle that helped us mediate against the psychic conflict between our superego and id. In *Myspace* and *Facebook*, the idea of a reality principle seems to get suspended indefinitely. *Myspace* and *Facebook* seem to have taken over where the video game *The Sims* left off. Chuck Klosterman describes *The Sims* in *Sex Drugs and Cocoa Puffs:*

> *The Sims* is a keenly constructed product that seems hopelessly absurd to anyone unfamiliar with it but completely clear to anyone who's experienced it even once. Developed by Electronic Arts, *The Sims* is a video game where you do all the things you would do in real life if you weren't playing a video game. You create a human character, and it exists. That's it. Your character does things like read the newspaper. He takes naps, plays pinball, and empties the garbage. Your character invites friends over to his house, and they have discussions about money and sailboats. You buy oak bookcases and you get a pizza from Domino's. This is the whole game, and there is no way to win, except to keep yourself from becoming depressed. *The Sims* is an escapist vehicle for people who want to escape to where they already are...
>
> (Klosterman 2003:13)

Instead of playing a person in the video game *The Sims*, you now can create and control your own ego and friends in *Myspace* and *Facebook*. You can control your looks, likes, style, interests, and desires without any checks and balances, like *The Sims*. The old Freudian idea of ego, which was part of the mind that mediated the conflicts of the conscious and unconscious mind and worked on a reality principle, has been completely abandoned. Our modern idea of ego fits beautifully in its place. *Myspace* and *Facebook* allow us to build our own ego and see how the world will react all while keeping track of friends like points.

Myspace and *Facebook* can allow users to test how others will think of their likes, thoughts, or style in the anonymity of cyber space and experience the pleasures of acknowledgement from another person without the risk of actual human interaction in the "real" world we live in. Or it allows you to be or act like someone you have always wanted to be, as you would while playing *The Sims*. Just as in playing the videogame

The Sims, your own ego doesn't have to bear the brunt of public scrutiny. You can try your new role or persona out from the safety of your own bedroom. The question to ask is how is you're *Myspace* or *Facebook* profile different from how you act in public? The reality of friends that you contact and have met only through a computer distort what it means to have friends that you talk to in person. Even your intimate friends in your everyday life are changed when you interact via a non-human form of communication. There is no replacement for exchanging ideas with another human being in their presence. Semioticians claim that between 66 percent 93 percent of our interactions with each other are done non-verbally (Miller 2000:7). This means even if you get everything on the page that you want, the meaning can be completely changed without the non-verbal message that would accompany the interaction in person. We need to be aware of the alterations that occur as we make "contact" more and more only through media technology. *Myspace* and *Facebook* are further portals of the media matrix that has altered our view of reality. The name is very appropriate for the culture that invented the "Me" Generation. Thirty years of exposure has impacted our psyche and ego even more profoundly and turned us into the "My" Generation where *Myspace* and *Facebook* are lonely places.

In the next chapter, we explore in detail our childhood relationship to television, and we see how television comes to life as a sort of wraparound, commercialized ghetto that tends to organize the very texture of our childhood life.

6
CHILDREN'S TV
Saturday Morning Ghetto

One aspect of television distinguishes it from all other past technologies that have affected society. No other advance had ever affected the lives of children under the age of six—the most impressionable segment of the population—as swiftly, pervasively, and directly as the coming of television to the American home.

(Winn 2002:283)

We'd like to begin this chapter regarding children's television by contrasting Marshall McLuhan's vision of media light with Marie Winn's vision of media darkness. In a 1969 *Playboy* interview, Marshall McLuhan gave a decidedly positive and optimistic endorsement of television as a truly educational force:

PLAYBOY: If you had children young enough to belong to the TV generation, how would you educate them?

MCLUHAN: Certainly not in our current schools, which are intellectual penal institutions. In today's world, to paraphrase Jefferson, the least education is the best education, since very few young minds can survive the intellectual tortures of our educational system. The mosaic image of the TV screen generates a depth-involving *nowness* and simultaneity in the lives of children that makes them scorn the distant visualized goals of traditional education as unreal, irrelevant and puerile ... . We have to ask what TV can do, in the instruction of English or physics or any other subject, that the classroom cannot do as presently constituted. *The answer is that TV can deeply involve youth in the process of learning,* illustrating graphically the complex interplay of people and events, the development of forms, the multileveled interrelationships between and among such arbitrarily segregated subjects as biology, geography, mathematics, anthropology, history, literature and languages.

(McLuhan and Zingrone 1995:251; second emphasis mine)

Eight years later in 1977, Marie Winn, in her groundbreaking, critical study on television as a plug-in drug, offered us a much-more skeptical, darker vision of "educational TV":

It is easy to overlook a deceptively simple fact: one is always watching television when one is watching television rather than having any other experience. Whether the program is Sesame Street or Batman, Reading Rainbow, or The Flintstones, there's a similarity of experience about all television watching. Certain specific physiological mechanisms of the eyes, ears, and brain respond to the stimuli emanating from the television screen regardless of the cognitive content of the programs.?

(Winn 2002:3)

The Media-Infused Classroom

"What is your earliest memory of television?" we asked our college media class one day. "How do you think watching television has actually affected your life? How has it affected your relationship to yourself, to the world and to other people? What is your media history? What does your personal media biography look like?" We were seeking to situate ourselves in an inquiry: We wanted to get at the dawn of conscious memory (or even unconscious memory) regarding our relationship with television. From there, we could explore and track the weaving, texture, and designs in the fabric of that relationship down through our life and mind. We wanted to pursue an "archaeological dig," as it were, on our buried, layered-over socialization process as it took shape in the presence of television. We wanted to look at our relationship to television *as a parental relationship*. To do this, we also used a sort of "koan-guided" inquiry: "Where does TV end and myself begin?" "Where do my parents end and my self begin?" We subdivided our archaeological dig into a number of exercises. The instructions for the overall exercise are, in a sense, quite simple: (1) Now that you are an adult, go back and watch children's television; (2) interview a young child about his or her current experience of television; and (3) visit a children's toy store with television in the foreground of your mind.

Marie Winn's Addiction Television

Winn's now classic book, *The Plug- in Drug*, is a deeply disturbing and disillusioning look at the actual effects of television on children. Fetal alcohol syndrome is a truly tragic experience and also a devastatingly damning consequence deriving from the behavior of the parent of the newborn infant. In a somewhat analogous way (children television syndrome), the television drug can be seen as deeply damaging, both mentally and socially. It is a plug-in-drug that parents often inflict on their children to pacify, control, and occupy them—which is not unlike the view that it is a drug that governments, ruling orders, inflict upon their populations to pacify, control, and occupy them.

> *Erica:* I am truly part of the television generation...My most vivid memory of my childhood was television. The television in many ways was my best friend. When I was lonely I turned the television on and it made me feel not so alone. To this day the television keeps me company when I feel alone. Watching television has become a habit for me. When I come home, I automatically turn the box on, regardless if I'm watching it or not, I just like it on. I like to do my homework when it is on, or eat dinner; I even like to fall asleep when it is on.
>
> I see this happening with my younger brother. He is only four years old but he knows how to operate the VCR as well as get access to all the cable channels. He has a collection of fifty video cartoon movies and watches them over and over...
>
> We lost my brother to the television. He gets entranced by it and is lost in the make believe world the television has created for him. I look at my brother and it is like looking at myself at that age and even now. We both react the same. We both hear nothing else than what is on the show and block out the world around us. To give credit to my mother and stepfather, they do spend time with the both of us, but I couldn't get rid of my television if I wanted to. With the television on I'm not alone and I do not have to feel like I'm alone. This box has a powerful hold over

me. In many ways it is like a drug, a little is better than nothing. It has become an addiction for me as for many others.

In the context of our commercial media culture, people *use* TV much the same way as people *use* drugs and alcohol. In the process of documenting, exploring, and analyzing the addiction of children to television, Marie Winn makes a devastating observation: She notes that it is not the children who are the primary television addicts; rather, it is their parents. It is the parents, fatigued both by their own demanding life and by the incessant demands and energies of their children, who set them in front of the television screen. The television addiction is thus connected in *The Plug-In Drug* to the malfunctioning of the family. Television is often a drug administered by parents to their own children to make them quiet and docile because, in the short run, that seems easier than dealing with the children themselves.

Lisa: I started by asking my boyfriend about his media history. His first memory of TV was from before he was six years old. He remembers crawling out of his room with a blanket to sneak out and watch a TV game show. In his household, television was a babysitter. It was always there even when no one else was. His family always watched the news at dinner time. He said that they always knew what was happening in the world but not in each other's lives. Television played a moderately big role in his life during his younger years. TV was a good friend … . The next person I spoke to was Dave's sister Suzanne. Although they grew up in the same house, their TV habits were very different. She was always watching TV and it was always on whether or not she was paying direct attention to it. She used to cut school in order to watch General Hospital. She said that she really couldn't remember when the TV wasn't on and available. It seems as though their entire family togetherness was based on watching television. Even now when we (Dave and I) go to visit his parents and sister at their home, there is always someone watching the TV. And for the most part, we spend our time visiting, or rather, watching TV together.

I watched a tremendous amount of TV as a kid. Way too much. I remember when my parents would go out for the evening, they would allow me to stay up an extra half hour to watch more TV. It was a reward for me. I also remember eating all of my meals in front of the TV. We never had family dinners until I was in college and even then, the TV was on and everyone could see it from the table. That seems kind of weird to me now but it has definitely carried over into my adult life. I would still rather watch TV while I eat rather than sit at the dining room table and make conversation. It is almost as though I am socially dysfunctional at times because of the TV. I wasn't taught those skills as a kid. The TV taught me how to interact--or not to. I am kind of angry that TV played such a big part in my growing up years. I definitely consider myself a television junkie, a TV-aholic, and I am finding it very difficult to give it up cold turkey. They should have TV Watchers Anonymous … . The more I learn, the more I want to bomb my TV set. I'm just not sure how I would live without it.

One of the main aspects of Winn's argument is that *children experience television very differently than do adults.* Children have no horizon of life-experience upon which to situate what they see on the television *as television*; hence, the television experience itself becomes the horizon of life. "For surely the hours that children spend in a one-way relationship with television people, an involvement that allows for no communication or interaction must have some effect on their relationships with real-life people." (Winn 2002:158). For the most part, adults see television in the context of life. Children have not yet developed that context, and hence they are overwhelmingly at the mercy of seeing television as life. As they have no deep anchorage in reality against which to experience television, television itself tends to become their anchorage in reality. In the presence of TV, children are, as it were, hyper-gullible.

Patricia: As a family, we would watch the latest episode of Lassie. I have early memories of watching the show and becoming so involved with the unfolding drama that I would yell at the television set. "Watch out, Timmy! Be careful, Lassie! RUN, LASSIE, RUN!!" would tumble out of my excited and worried mouth. The emotion of watching a stressful episode would sometimes be too much that I would hide under a table and watched the scary scene from between my fingers. I would stay under the table until I felt that any eminent danger portrayed was finally over. I later came to realize that if something really bad were to happen to Lassie, the television series would end and there would be no show the following week. Subconsciously, I gradually began to watch Lassie with less emotional investment. I guess it was at that point that I became a little jaded…

For the infant human animal, seeing is believing. In the beginning of our television watching, television doesn't have "entertainment value." In the beginning, television is *not* entertainment. It's real. Later we transform it into "entertainment."

The electronic companionship dimension of TV teaching is profound and runs deep yet is often overlooked. Winn argues that television is used as a babysitter by parents, or rather that television is misused and overused as a babysitter. If TV is first experienced as our third parent, it obviously has deep repercussions down the corridors of time as we use it throughout our life. If our childhood, imprint experience of TV is as an electronic babysitter, a surrogate electronic parent, most likely all our future experiences of it, however diverse, adult, and sophisticated they may be, will happen inside that primary imprint. They will happen on the horizon of that primary, indelible family experience established in our childhood. We may be watching the news, but nevertheless we are subliminally *in the presence of companionship*. We subconsciously experience ourselves related to the television in the mode of personal companionship. Children are *bonding* with television characters and with programs.

The Horizon of Television

There is a certain horizon of reality that TV culture promotes—an endless in-the-distance-phenomenon that we are journeying toward and aspiring to. This horizon of reality becomes the background against which we experience and evaluate our own lives and the lives of others. This background phenomenon has deep implications for the objects, persons, and experiences that we experience on the foreground.

TV and the culture it anchors have now become the horizon of reality that guides our way of being-in-the-world. It has become that transcendent ground upon which we experience our experience. It outlines the very texture of what it is that we experience. *It is not itself a discreet experience but it enframes all our discrete experiences.* Somewhat analogous to how the Catholic Church was the horizon of experience in the European Medieval Age—permeating and resonating all through the texture of life, inner life and outer life—so commercial television culture now soaks through all our experiences. Our lives, or more precisely, our reflections on and representations of our lives, have been marinated in commercial television.

If television culture provides the horizon of reality of our envisioned life, we are in television—*in* television, not watching television, not on television, but inside television. Inside the cave, somewhere in our subterranean depths, we expect our life to be like the lives we see on television. When our life does not seem to be happening according to these expectations, we don't abandon the expectations: That's like making the horizon disappear. We look to see how we can "fix things" so that it comes into line with the televised world. The nature of this "fixing" is almost always related to consuming-buying.

Instructions for Saturday Morning Ghetto Exercise

The instructions for this exercise were, as we said earlier, quite simple: Watch children's television, interview a child about television, and visit a toy store. Let us spell out in a bit more detail each of these instructions.

1. In terms of watching children's television, the specific instructions were to watch any commercial television show on Saturday morning that is specifically intended for children. Then, in contrast, watch any non-commercial children's show—mostly this will be PBS or possibly cable. The intent here is to become more precisely aware of the difference between commercial and non-commercial children's television, especially in reference to the values and ways of seeing the world that are woven into the fabric of the show. The *Saturday morning ghetto* is a term intended to highlight the cluster of values broadcast by the commercial media that is specifically directed at children. This is, thus, a study in media child psychology.

2. In terms of interviewing a child about *their* experience of watching television, we told our students that we wanted them to really *get into the child's world.* As we said earlier, the TV is *not* "TV" to

children. The challenge in this inquiry was to abandon the self-evident dimensions of the adult's experience of TV and allow oneself to venture inside the child's world, to submit somehow to the magic of this childhood experience.

3. The adventure or expedition into the toy store was to be undertaken both as an anthropological journey into an uncharted and strange land and as an archaeologist's discovery of the artifacts of a lost civilization. We all grew up with our toys, and almost all of us went to toy stores as children. Here the challenge was to de-familiarize oneself with the concept of "toy" and "toy store" as we have come to think about them as adults. Along with the archaeologist analogy, we also suggested that students do this with the context of cultural anthropology's field ethnographer in mind: Approach going into the toy store as if you were entering a foreign, alien, strange, and unknown culture—because, in fact, your are! Pay attention to the physical design of the store, the architectural space, the messages and intentions that are built into that space, that are folded and tucked into those display-arrangements. A secondary dimension to this undertaking was to pay particular attention to the *gender curriculum* that is built into the toy store. See what you can see.

Angela: As I walked into Toys'R'Us I felt nauseous. There were so many bright colors, crammed shelves and things hanging from the ceiling that I was overwhelmed. I can only imagine how a child would react in such an environment... I strolled up and down the isles and saw the most awesome toys. Where were all these toys when I was little? I picked two toys that looked appealing to me and investigated the boxes. I saw that I had both dolls when I was younger and neither one were worth the money. It was the packaging that made the dolls look so appealing. It was all advertising. There was just tons and tons of advertising around me. 38 isles. 13 feet high of pure ads. Worthless, useless, cheap toys packaged brilliantly.

   I studied a little boy for a couple of minutes and noticed he was begging, screaming, and crying how he'd wanted this rocket toy forever. His mother sternly said "no" and within seconds he had jumped to a different toy that he'd desperately needed before he'd switched his mind to another, and then again; just like changing channels with a remote control. As his mom got more and more pissed, she yelled to her son "Go see if they have a TV you can watch." This was the most brilliant piece of knowledge I have heard all semester.

After returning to my house, I browsed over my notes and little by little began to see the connection between the toy store and television. Toys play off TV and TV plays off toys, using colorful, chaotic ads to suck the children in. Then when a child is in the store, the ad begins to sell the toy. Immediately I saw our society cramming its views into the toy store. The majority of toys in the girls department were dolls. White dolls. Tall, thin, blond haired, blue eyed dolls. The boys department had guns, guns, and more guns, tanks, fire engines and police cars, anything that represented war, total chaos and control.

What is the overall purpose of this Saturday morning ghetto exercise? It provides access to an ordinary environment in a perspicuous manner—which is to say, it allows us to see usual and familiar things in a provocative and unusual manner. This unusual manner of seeing usual things thrusts us into the space of critical inquiry, of questioning that which we wouldn't ordinarily question or even notice for that matter. The purpose of this exercise is to cease seeing television shows in their natural environment of passive, spectator absorption and to put them into an environment of attentiveness, an environment of "contrast and compare" attentiveness. A number of techniques and ideas are compressed in this endeavor: First, we are paying attention to the television show, rather than watching it. We get instant access here to the phenomenon that to watch TV is *not* to pay attention to it. Second, we are somewhat revisiting shows that for the most part we have already been quite familiar with as children. There is a sense of traveling back in time to our childhood world, yet with the mind of an adult—an interesting blend. The really difficult, personal, and profound question here is "Does watching TV as a child have any *continuing effect* on me as an adult?" Third, we are engaged in a compare-and-contrast mode of inquiry. By juxtaposing two items next to each other, we get to see a third "item" that wasn't present when we viewed each item separately and compartmentally. Finally, we are to some degree lifting a trap door at the ground floor level of our adult reality and peeking underneath to catch a glimpse of the magical realm of children's television. We should add, the magical realm on the *receiving end* of children's television, for along with this also comes critical insight into the disturbing, exploitive, *producing, and transmitting end* of children's television.

Interview a Pre-Schooler

We would like in this section to simply let our students speak without our commentary.

Shannon: Interviewing a three-year-old was frustrating. When I asked him if he ever watched Sesame Street he said he watched it every morning (which was confirmed by the day care supervisor) and yet when asked what kinds of things he learns or what kinds of things are talked about on Sesame Street he had no idea. His exact words were, "I don't learn anything. I just watch."

Watching this child was like watching a television. He was TV personified. His actions, his speech, the games he liked to play, his opinions, and in some way his identity, all seemed derived from and manufactured by TV.

Patricia: Malcolm is a 3-year-old boy who loves to play with his Thomas and Friends train set which is based on the children's show Thomas and Friends. He showed me his trains and I enthusiastically said, "Oh wow! Let's play!" ... . Malcolm told a lot of stories about the different train characters while he was playing with them. It was as if he was narrating his own play. This is very interesting, as the children's show Thomas and Friend uses the same format of a voice-over storyteller to narrate each episode. I couldn't get a clear answer as to whether or not Malcolm's stories were his own inventions or his reiteration of something he remembered from watching television. The fact that he was narrating his own play indicated to me that the storytelling format used on the television show impresses 3-year-old Malcolm greatly.

Alice: From the day my little brother came home from the hospital I have been helping to take care of him; in a way he grew up having two moms. When he was little we would always play together. I could spend hours with him and not notice the time pass by, but now that feeling is not being reciprocated.

He has found television, and it is his new best friend. He still loves to play with his toys and loves his friends, but television is one of his top priorities. He started out watching basketball with his dad, and he liked it because the players in their bright uniforms were constantly on the move. He slowly graduated from basketball to watching Barney and Sesame Street. He never watched too often though, and it did not encompass his entire life. However, he started to become more active, and my mom, who works full time, needed a break from all of his energy. She gradually let him watch more and more television until finally my stepfather was upset because my brother's television watching was interfering with his own viewing time. My mom gave in and bought a television for my brother's room. This is when my brother's life began to change.

He now needs television. He will sit there for hours watching anything that flashes by the screen, and the fact that there are cartoons on twenty-four hours a day does not help. He can be a very sweet and caring little boy when he is not being drugged by television, but John gets very upset, almost angry if you try to talk to him while he is watching. I have gone in to say good-bye to him when I am leaving for school, but if he is watching a cartoon he will merely ask me to leave because I am bothering him. He has been completely taken in by this little flashing box.

The remote control seems to be his life link. At nighttime he stays awake watching cartoons and finally falls asleep with the remote tightly clutched in his little hand. If the remote is removed at all he jumps up searching for it, and it has to be there when he first wakes up in the morning. When I was young I had a blanket that I thought kept me safe, but John has an electronic device that provides no warmth and comfort at all. My mom insists that he does not watch too much television. Her rationale is that he deserves a break in the evening since he is in school all day. I can see her point of view because she works all day and does not have the energy to entertain my little brother when she gets home. I just wish that he could spend some time without it or at least remove it from his bedroom. I know this will never happen. It has now become a necessity for both my brother and my parents. When I asked John about television I was surprised by his answers.

To John, everything that appears on television is real. He knows that cartoons are different from real people, but he was not quite sure how they were different.

Emilia: When living with a younger child, it seems like it is nearly impossible to get any work done when they are in your presence. They want you to "play with them" or "read them a book" or "take them to a park"—don't they understand that you have things you NEED to get done?! My little sister never seemed to understand that. So, what was my solution? Turn on the TV to any cartoon I could find and sit her down in front of it. Problem solved. She was being entertained, as long as it wasn't by me, and I was able to get done what needed to be done. As years passed, I began to notice that my sister spent most of her day watching the TV. What was the first thing she did when she got home from school? Turn on the TV immediately. My mom would have to yell at her to go wash up for a snack and most of the time my sister ignored her. My sister had become addicted to TV. And as I notice this problem, I couldn't help but feel I was partly to blame. After all, my sister was being deprived of her imagination, her creativity, her intellect--all because my family and I chose to let the TV replace those things. TV does nothing for children, except provide meaningless entertainment and a false perception of reality.

As I began to notice how much more my sister was watching TV, I also noticed her attention span toward us was decreasing while her attention span for the TV was increasing. It was so bad that I could walk into the living room where she was watching the television, say something to her, and be completely ignored. She was so captivated by what she was watching on the TV screen that she didn't even notice that I had said something to her …

Play Deprivation

Play is the child's royal road to intelligence, creative thinking, and joy. The child who can play will play skillfully and successfully throughout life.

(Mendizza and Pearce 2003:ix).

There are, according to Winn, deep reverberations for those who have spent a majority of their childhood watching instead of playing.   If children spend every waking hour watching television instead of creating a game, using their imaginations, or even socializing, they will go through "play deprivation." Play deprivation can effect the primary tone of joy or depression one may have towards life itself. As the researcher Brian Sutton-Smith wrote in his "Children at Play" article for the journal, Natural History

> The primary purpose of play has a deeper importance for every individual. Playing children are motivated primarily to enjoy living. This is the major rehearsal value of play and games, for without the ability to enjoy life, the long years of adulthood can be dull and wearisome.
>
> (Sutton-Smith 1971:59)

Too much childhood television and not enough childhood play can lead to a person's inability to enjoy life. When children play they learn to make the best out of any situation. Those who know how to create games and make laborious work fun are the ones who can enjoy life to its fullest. Those who have a need for continuous entertainment, provided by outside forces, lack the skills to make and to create seemingly boring situations enjoyable on their own. They are thus more apt to fall into depressing states because it is hard for them to change their attitude and create other possibilities.

Saturday Morning TV

There is a metaphysical dualism, a basic premise of life, deeply embedded in the teachings of Saturday morning cartoons: good versus evil. As television children, we are overwhelmingly and unambiguously taught that the central axis around which life turns is good defeating evil, heroes defeating villains. This teaching is as visible in the demagogical posturing of our adult presidents during times of crises and wars— President Reagan's posturing towards the Soviet Union as "the evil empire," the posturing by both Presidents Bush toward Saddam Hussein as the arch villain and the "axis of evil"—as it is in children's cartoons. We are trained first to see the world and its operations in terms of good versus evil, and then we are trained to see ourselves as the good guys. To believe in and feel ourselves as "the good guy," we *must have* an "evil villain" *to oppose* and *fight against*. This becomes the basic drama of life: pure good against complete evil (Nietzsche 1967). The cartoon characters are also super-human and visibly heroic in their abilities and actions. The commercial products in the advertisements aimed at children are also displayed as having exaggerated, "heroic" abilities, and hence the commercial products by association become super-human and heroic.

> *Lisa:*   Children's programming on major commercial networks broadcast many cartoons that are violent and that distort reality. The characters in these cartoons are fictitious and are shown performing super-natural heroic acts. The basic premise of these cartoons is heroes against villains. The shows depict good guys always catching the bad guys. The characters are stereotypical in nature, meaning that they are either good or evil. Characters like teenage mutant ninja turtles, or scooby doo, are often shown flipping through the air and running faster than the speed of light. Children see their heroic abilities on television and at a young age are unable to differentiate between fiction and fantasy. The same goes for commercials, which portray products in a manipulative manner, which exaggerates the products abilities and functions. Children's television is basically propaganda. I was surprised to see so much use of violence and sexual innuendos by the media in cartoons and by advertisers to sell products.

Once you begin to live in an imaginary world where the basic dramatic function of your life is to fight evil, your own motive system is sealed off and secured. You never have to examine the roots of your own behavior and actions (Nietzsche 1967). The focus of attention is never on what motivates the good guys but rather what evil wickedness must be fought and triumphed over. "Us verses them" is always deeply soothing and satisfying in its unequivocal military simplicity: I need never look into my self, my reasons, my existence; my job is to fight evil, period.

TV, Toys, and Attachment

> *Jane:*   I visited the famous Toys'R'Us. I was intrigued from the moment I walked in. It was like I had just entered into the TV screen in my living room … . They had any kind of toy that I could imagine, or, rather that the TV could imagine for me.

The children of today are constantly persuaded by the media, mainly television, to acquire more and more possessions. These television-associated possessions, mainly toys, limit a child's ability to imagine and create a plethora of worlds and scenarios during their playtime. This is owing to the fact that a teenage mutant ninja turtle transport bus can do only that which it is designed to do. It is also designed for the purpose of creating the desire to own more ninja turtle toys to accompany it. Only ninja turtles can fit into a ninja turtle bus. Toys of the past, such as Legos, tinker toys, and other wooden objects, were more open-ended toward the horizon of creativity and imaginativeness. Simple toys allowed for children to imagine many worlds, subject to change as the child so chose. Many plastic toys tend to pre-create, as it were, the child's world of imagination. Couple this with the fact that children watch an average of 27 hours per week of TV programming geared toward the main objective of selling them more plastic toys and you begin to see a very powerful phenomenon.

The firewall between reality and the world of fictional TV and video games is erased in toy stores. The hyper, warp-speed world of media dominates the atmosphere as the big, bright, plastic toys that have lots of buttons to push are easily "chosen" or "wanted" over a box of Legos. Children now are conditioned into choosing a created world, an *already* created world, rather than a world allowing them to be creative and to create. They are conditioned to want to be entertained by something rather than developing entertainment for themselves. On some level, children are losing the ability to think and act independently of what TV creators create and, culturally speaking, dictate.

In regard to the toy-store-television connection, we think the most important thing to notice is the astonishing *presence* of TV *in* the toys. Once we wipe our commercial culture's advertising fairy dust from our eyes, it is a little disturbing what we see in a kid's toy store. It feels like we stepped into a living commercial set without cameras. The kid's sections of book stores have become similar. Toys teach consumerism better than anything else. They are the first experience kids have with the retail system. The toy store is organized to stimulate the feeling of having the fantasy world presented in commercials actually surrounding you. The highly crafted packaging for toys feels more or less like frozen TV advertisements. The store as a whole is not a store but rather an environmental wraparound advertisement. How much of the toy industry is now just *another ad* for a TV character? How much are TV characters just *another ad* for toys? Rather than creating their own fantasy world, children now are trying to recreate television programs with their toys and play.

Children's toys are TV come to life. "Television toys" allow children to live in their television worlds even after the television is turned off. The television world is no longer sealed off behind the screen. That which was on the screen is now in the room. Televisual illusions become real in this magical scenario. It's not so much that TV escapes into the real world of the home but rather that the real world of the home space becomes part of the landscape of TV-world. The presence of the TV characters and props are now three-dimensional. They are items we can put on and clothe ourselves with. We can robe and costume ourselves in television. This is a sort of material approximation to virtual reality. Children's TV has become "interactive," as it were, in the sense that now the child's world of make-believe, fantasy, and play is deeply if not totally infested with commercial television products and characters.

> *Alexandra:*   As far as the connection between toys and television, it is scary. For every toy on the shelf there is a corresponding television cartoon or action figure. After ten minutes of careful observation it is easy to see that television sells toys and toys sell television. The relationship is blatant and reciprocal. Kids watch TV to learn which toys to buy and then they go to the toy store to learn which TV programs to watch. It is a never-ending cycle.
>
> It was also apparent how rigid and defined the lines of gender are in our society. Walking through the store you could have basically built a barricade separating the female and male toys. It is indisputable by the walls of pink directly facing the towers of blue. As a child you must realize your place in the world and proceed accordingly to the corresponding display of gender-specific toys. We like to think that gender stereotyping is no longer prevalent in our society. If that is the case then why were all of the obviously 'boy toys' weapons and action figures, compared to the 'girl toys' like Barbie and pretend kitchen appliances? From the age of three we are teaching our women how to operate an E-Z Bake oven,

while our young men learn to recognize an AK-47. Surely some form of social control is at work here.

In reference to the gender curriculum and training principles built into the toys themselves, the values are genuinely destructive—either domesticator or terminator. The toy store is organized with little boys and girls in mind, but it has decided what the appropriate toys for each gender are supposed too be: The toys are packaged and marketed exclusively to only one gender or the other. There is an intense, humorless gender apartheid manufactured into the toys and the store. The block-headed, discriminating gender stereotyping that our society has come finally to condemn is nevertheless boldly taught at an early age and celebrated in the toy store. There are no pictures of girls playing with trucks or of boys playing with dolls. It has been set up in a way whereby children really do not get a choice in the kinds of toys that they like.

Patricia: As I went through the store I saw that all the aisles were color coded, with hot pink for all the girl toys and electric blue for all the boy toys. Even the pet aisle was separated by a pink side and a blue side! I saw very little in presentation, both in the way the store was organized or the packaging of toys that allowed for any gender overlapping. I also noticed that the majority of the name-brand toys were connected in some way to some sort of television or movie media, both commercial and non-commercial … . There were a lot of disturbing things that I saw in the store, but the most disgusting item I found was in the Princess Disney aisle. There I discovered a softball and softball bat set for girls that was covered with colorful images of Disney princesses. The ball was almost as soft as a hacky sac and the vinyl covered bat could not possibly carry any punch whatsoever. It was Disney's feeble attempt at creating a gender-balanced sport set. Here are a couple of messages I think the princess set conveyed: girls really don't want to play with this set because the set, like little girls, is too pretty to get dirty or sporty. Disney doesn't make real sports sets for girls because they will only hit a baseball like a girl anyway.

Children are being told how they should act, and any deviation from this is viewed as abnormal. So many of the boy's toys are powerfully hate-filled with a theme of either violence or masculine rhetoric inscribed all over them. They are really not made for little boys but for little soldiers. The sole purpose of much of the boy's toys is destruction. In the Saturday morning ghetto, the contrast between an action-packed world of violence and the dull ordinary world of human reality is visibly celebrated and reinforced. All the fun is in the fighting.

Where does TV end and the toy begin? What do toys teach? How is TV *in* the toy? What is the gender curriculum of the toy store? Looking at the toy store as the school, the university for children, we believe most parents would be surprised by what that curriculum teaches. Our children's toys today are *extensions* of television shows—there are almost no toys that stand on there own, so to speak—they are all related to TV. If the toy is an *extension* of the TV show, the child playing with it also becomes a *participant* in the TV show.

There is a visible, physical presence of television commercials all over the toy store. In fact, you can't really distinguish where the TV ends and the toy begins, as they are seamlessly continuous. Today's toys are made more and more out of a kind of television technology. You feel like you are walking into a peculiar sort of television land. The toy store becomes a sort of live cartoon you can walk into, and when you buy this toy, you are buying three-dimensional access to the TV show. With your toy, you know your place as a character in the show. The *magic and magical properties* of toys in the child's world are now completely interpenetrated with the magical qualities of television. Rather than using toys to magically invent and participate in a created world, children now choose an already pre-created and produced world—"as seen on TV." Toy manufacturers now create toys in *reference to TV*.

> *Jennifer:* Toys are now forced to compete with television for a child's attention … . Perhaps even more successful are those toys which could not exist without television. Sponge Bob toys are designed to make television a part of Sponge Bob fan's non-TV play time as are all other movie or TV themed playthings. [Notice that play is now often referred to as non-TV play.] A toy's function, then, is no longer to engage the child's own imagination, but to make someone else's imagination come to life.

This radical and subtle interpenetration of commercial media and child psychology has far reaching implications. Childhood characters

are no longer *just in* the TV world: All these characters have escaped
into Toy-world. There is a magical portal between the two worlds, and
the palpable, environmental, material presence of television media is
greatly re-enforced by the toy-object. With the toy, I hold a pulsating
piece of the television show in my hands. These toys are also layered
over with the quality of being props in the dramas of television. Given
all this, another subtle, almost undetectable level of realism is coated on
to our experience of television.

> *Patrick:* So where is it that the television ends and the toy begins? I
> think the answer is that the toy is an extension of the television. Another
> view is that the television itself is a toy. If we look at it, the TV is a very
> interactive game to a young child. You press a button and you see a picture.
> You press a different button and that picture goes away. Sounds like a toy
> to me. Lets look at the remote control. First of all, it is small enough for
> any child to play with. He can sit on the couch and hold it in his or her
> hands. It has buttons, which for a child constitutes something to play
> with. When the child pushes one of those buttons there is a response from
> another device. Constant pushing of buttons results in constant changes
> in the other devices behavior. Sounds like a game to me.
>
> So the answer of where the television ends and the toy begins is
> really redundant. It begins with the television and leads with the toy …
> When the child matures he will see the television as a media tool, but
> the element of a toy is still there. It is amazing that a plastic box can have
> so much power.

What is the problem with all this? Media imperialism. It colonizes
the child's world with commercial television. The fundamental concerns
of commercial television are now firmly embedded inside the hearts
and souls of children's toys. Who can overestimate the impact that our
childhood toys and games have upon us? Our toys and games are not
just toys and games. They are crucial to our forming ourselves. Children
play *very seriously*. There is a different quality to childhood play and
games than there is to adult play and games. Adults have the distinction
that it is "only" a game. There is no "only" in childhood play and games.
Childhood play and games are in some sense before, and even beyond,
the adult distinction of real or make believe. It is never "only" a game.

What are the fundamental concerns of commercial television? To push products for a profit. The crucial goal of all commercial programming is to seduce, shape, and reinforce the viewers into the consuming audience, that is, the audience who will consume the show—who will relate to the television show as a consumer product, which is to say as that to which we attach and addict. The intent is that the audience will consume the products advertised in and around the show and the show itself.

Commercial television is concerned with *attaching us to its fantasies*. The implications of this way of being run very deep: We attach to our show. We attach to our toys. We attach to our fantasies and our dreams. We attach to attaching to fantasy and make-believe. We come to believe in make-believe, in the efficacy and necessity of make-believe. Without fantasy and dreams and make-believe, *life is not worth living*, which is to say, *without television life is not worth living*. Recall the *TV Guide* poll we quoted in Chapter 5, "Would you swear of TV forever? For under one million bucks, no way. That's how nearly half of America's TV viewers feel. What's more, one-fourth of them wouldn't give it up even then."

The Lessons...

What are the central lessons to be learned from this exercise? The all-pervasive media world is all-pervasive. For childhood, *The Matrix* is indeed real. It exists in a sort of wraparound existentialism that organizes the very texture of our children's lives—and hence our adult lives as well for, as the old saying goes, "The child is father to the man."

The addiction quality is a central feature that emerges in our investigations of the media. Addiction, attachment, and dependency are organizations of our experience that happen again and again in almost every area of the media that we investigate: a fascination and fixation on the weightless experience of watching TV, a dependency and addiction, a craving quality that begins to grow and take hold, a drastic narrowing down of life to sitting and watching.

In the next chapter, we look in the mirror and seeing that we can no longer see ourselves clearly or simply but rather are haunted by advertisements from our commercial media.

7
Mirror TV
Looking Glass Self

On a daily basis, we see our reflection in the mirror as we groom ourselves. However, in our media age, we are not really *alone* when we see our reflection. If you want to see just how much you personally have been influenced by TV, just take a long, slow, 20-minute look in the mirror ... Do you see it? ... Do you see it inhabiting the way you see? ...

We see our reflection on the horizon of the television culture we have internalized. We don't so much see as we *evaluate* our reflected image. How does it compare to the images we have been drinking in for years from the other mirror, the television screen—that glowing mirror, ever radiating light, streaming forth an endless profusion of images? In our bathroom mirror, we see our reflection *not* in reference to ourselves. Rather, we see our reflection against the overwhelming host and teeming profusion of commercial representations. We can no longer really *be with* our reflection *alone*, in silence, with clarity in a non-judgmental, not-evaluative space.

We children of the television-parent are brought up and trained to judge ourselves in comparison with the beautiful and perfect media parent people. That is a large reason why having negative feelings about our physical appearance is so very, very common among us.

> One of the things that makes the people on television fit to stand the Megagaze is that they are, by ordinary human standards, extremely pretty. I suspect that this, like most television conventions, is set up with no motive more sinister than to appeal to the largest possible Audience— pretty people tend to be more appealing to look at than non-

pretty people. But when we're talking about television, the combination of sheer Audience size and quiet psychic intercourse between images and oglers starts a cycle that both enhances pretty people's appeal and erodes us viewers' own security in the face of gazes. Because of the way human beings relate to narrative, we tend to identify with those characters we find appealing. We try to see ourselves in them. The same I.D.-relation, however, also means that we try to see them in ourselves. When everybody we seek to identify with for six hours a day is pretty, it naturally becomes more important to us to be pretty, to be viewed as pretty. Because prettiness becomes a priority for us, the pretty people on TV become all the more attractive, a cycle which is obviously great for TV. But it's less great for us civilians, who tend to own mirrors, and who also tend not to be anywhere near as pretty as the TV-images we want to identify with. Not only does this cause some angst personally, but the angst increases because, nationally, everybody else is absorbing six-hour doses and identifying with pretty people and valuing prettiness more, too. This very personal anxiety about our prettiness has become a national phenomenon with national consequences…It's not paranoid or hysterical to acknowledge that television in enormous doses affects people's values and self-perception in deep ways. Nor that televisual conditioning influences the whole psychology of one's relation to himself, his mirror, his loved ones, and a world of real people and real gazes.

(Wallace 1997:53)

We once asked our students in several classes to raise their hands if they had ever been on a diet. *All* of the women had been on diets. Some of the men had, even though the only even slightly overweight body in those rooms belonged to a young man who said that he had thought about it but never actually did it. Women are taught to set more store by their appearance than men. Men act, women appear, as the old adage goes. Men are taught to overlook and disattend to their appearance more than women. And somehow, no matter how many diets we embark on or how many cosmetics and exercise machines we buy, *we remain imperfect.* Anxiety about non-perfection becomes obsessional within our televisual culture.

This is because, unlike the media beauties, we are real people. Most people don't realize the outrageous extent to which media beauties are made up, carefully lighted, sometimes even sewn into their clothes to a point that looks good but would make actual movement impossible. But that is just the beginning. After being filmed or photographed, the picture is altered through various techniques to hide imperfections and create a certain "mood." Photography technicians and commercial graphic artists have been known to put one person's head on another person's body.

Cindy Crawford, a fashion model, has been quoted saying she wished she looked like the Cindy Crawford in the magazines.

> Photogenic beauty rests its definition of perfection on a smooth, standardized, and lifeless modernism, a machine aesthetic in the guise of a human. Caught in time it is a perfection that never ages, and experiences no mood swings. . . Even for those - mostly women - whose faces and bodies provide the raw materials for these images, comparisons are invidious. Against the flat, clichéd view of reality that they portray in the fashion photograph, all elements of lived experience constitute potential flaws ... . *beautiful thinghood* becomes an affliction; the image of self stirs painful feelings of inadequacy. In a 1986 television interview, singer/actress Lanie Kazan spoke revealingly of a seven-year period of crisis, during which she fell victim to the corroding influence of her own publicity photos. Haunted by her inability to live up to, or embody, the air-brushed perfection of the image, she became housebound. "I went to bed in 1969," she related, "and didn't get up until 1976 ... . I would not go out until I looked like my photograph."
>
> (Ewen 1988:89)

In an experiment wherein women were shown ads featuring beautiful models while another group was shown the same ads that featured only a picture of the product, it was found that the women who had been shown the models didn't particularly want the products measurably more but did become measurably more critical of their own appearances than those who had seen the ads without the models. Women's self-esteem drops after looking at beauty images for just a few moments.

A poignant story is told by Gloria Steinem about Eleanor Roosevelt. She was a homely, shy child, yet she became the most powerful woman in America as the first lady. Her husband, Franklin Roosevelt, really listened to her and supported her countless activities on behalf of the underdog. After his death, she served at the United Nations and became perhaps the most widely respected woman in the world. Yet, when asked if she had any regrets about her life, she said, "Just one. I wish I'd been prettier" (Steinem 1993:226). What man in her position would have felt that way?

Most women have negative body images. At the same time that feminism has won some legal and economic advances, especially for middle-class women, there has been a concomitant rise in the media emphasis on the importance of replicating media versions of beauty. Plastic surgeons have never had so much business. Naomi Wolf, in discussing contemporary women, observes that "… in terms of how we feel about ourselves *physically*, we may actually be worse off than our unliberated grandmothers" (Wolf 1991:10).

There is little connection between having a negative image and actual appearance. However, there is, thanks to media, a strong connection between body image and self-esteem. The way to genuine self-esteem is not, we hold, through attempting to change one's appearance. It is rather a process of seeing through media-unreality and rejecting this humiliating view of us as human beings whose comparative and competitive outsides are more important than our insides, our minds and hearts.

Unfortunately, the media have made this connection between self-esteem and body image so ubiquitous, so tangible, that for many individuals, cosmetic surgery seems to be the only answer to feeling whole and complete. It is better in the minds of these individuals to surgically alter their bodies than not fit into the mold created by the media. There have been numerous shows in the media about people changing their bodies and looks through surgery, not to mention the celebrities who flaunt their modifications. Most of these shows are sensational and powerful in the transformation that takes place in the look of the person or people featured. One especially cruel version of these shows pitted individuals with severe self-esteem issues about their looks in a beauty pageant after going through complete cosmetic surgery makeover of their entire bodies. Even after a complete alteration, only one of these individuals left being told they were the winner. What can be done for the self-esteem of the other contestants when you have completely changed your body and face to fit the media's mold and still are not good enough? Regardless of the show, the prominent existence of them in the media give more credence to the idea of modifying our bodies to fit this unrealistic media mold.

In the last year, there were over 10 million cosmetic procedures in the United States, ranging from the non-surgical Botox and laser hair removal to surgically invasive breast augmentation and rhinoplasty (boob and nose jobs). According to the Web site of the *American Society for Aesthetic Plastic Surgery*, there has been a 457 percent increase of cosmetic procedures and a 743 percent increase of non-surgical procedures since 1997 (when they began collecting their statistics). Is the substantial rise in the number of these cosmetic procedures and there prevalence in the media a coincidence? We don't believe so; in a sense, these shows have created a new consumer beauty product: *ourselves.* Instead of using makeup or other beauty aides, now we buy ourselves whatever we feel will make us look and feel better by changing our bodies. Undergoing surgery to change our appearance is often a form of self-abuse that makes it harder, not easier, to come to a comfortable, accepting relationship with our self. Men have also been hit by media images. Many have also acquired negative opinions about their bodies, but the phenomenon is much greater in women. For men, not living up to the media stereotype involves wanting to be taller and more muscular and wanting a more impressive penis (Steinem 1993:221–229).

It may help us all to realize that fashions in appearance differ from culture to culture or from one historical epoch to another. When you look at the female nudes cavorting about on Rubens' huge, nineteenth-century canvasses, what you see would make the diet industry salivate with glee: They are all "fat ladies" by our present standards. Yet, interestingly enough, studies in evolutionary psychology show women as different-looking as Venus di Milo, Marilyn Monroe, and Kate Moss share the same hip-to-waist ratio.

The Looking Glass Self: From the Familiar Stranger to the Empty Mirror

We see our face the way we do not because that's the way it is but because we have these ways of seeing. We all think, quite unproblematically, that we know what we look like. In terms of common sense, if someone asked us whether we knew what we looked like, we would respond,

"Of course, we know what we look like." It is precisely the "*of-course*" dimensions of our life that have been one of the major concerns of sociology. We've seen our reflection in the mirror hundreds, thousands of times. Nothing new there—nothing unknown or unfamiliar. Insofar as a large dimension of the sociological perspective is to de-familiarize the all too familiar world, to see not exotic, new things but rather old familiar things in new ways, an investigation into our familiar image might prove to be very fruitful and provocative—especially in reference to its relation to the commercial mass media.

In this section, we explore the mirror. We might discover the shocking degree to which we habitually *don't* see what's there, what's literally there. We don't see our self as we are, now; we are always looking ahead to how we will be perceived ... by others. We *project rather than perceive*. In reference to our socialization process, this entire exercise is really about seeing ourselves as we are and not as we have been conditioned to want to be. Hence, one result is that we see the alarming and unsettling degree to which the symbolic world created by the social institution of media, especially advertising, is now deeply, subcutaneously, inside us. We might discover that our own personal views and feelings toward our image have long ago been quietly supplanted. We might discover, especially in the pain of our critical self-hatred, that we are now carriers of this advertising culture, trained and preoccupied with self-rejection rather than self-acceptance, trained to over-identify with commercial judgments of ourselves and others. "Where does advertising end and my self begin?" Another result we may discover is the radical degree to which we can't in fact see what others see when they see us. We can't see ourselves in the way that others see us. In this sense, we are forever invisible to ourselves. (This, interestingly enough, may prove to be a liberating experience from the earlier depressions and imprisonments we may encounter.)

The Instructions We Gave Our Students

1. Observe your face in the mirror *for 20 minutes*. See what you can see. Or, perhaps, see what you see. Don't *do* anything. Resist the habit of the mirror. Just be there. In reference to your mind, do not daydream, drift off, or fantasize. Do not engage-yourself-in-

remembering-your-past-nor-in-planning- your-future. Be present, aware and precise. As best you can, do this exercise with "beginner's mind."

2. Strip down and look at yourself in the mirror for 10 minutes *as naked* (without clothes) and then again for 10 minutes *as nude* (without clothes but with an awareness of being seen by an imaginary other).

3. Go 24 hours without looking at your reflection in any mirror whatsoever. Cold-turkey.

What is the purpose of this exercise? To see our self. To see the non-substantiality of our self, the absence of a tangible thing. Our relationship with our reflection is indeed charged, complex, and endless. The seduction and fascination of the TV is perhaps minor in comparison to the seduction of the mirror. The familiar "that's me," for this experiment, seems to be both the experience and the problem.

From the perspective of asking "Where does the media end and my self begin?" the mirror offers an inescapable labyrinth of ambiguity, an inexhaustible series of feints, anxieties, and uncertainties. The uncertainty of the mirror mirrors the uncertainty of our relation to the Other: The primordial unpredictability, the indefinitely uncertain, the never-still, ever-unfolding unknownness and precariousness of inhabiting a world with Others—the intimate, the stranger, the relative, the friend, the enemy, the us, the them, the contemporaries, the predecessors, the descendants—the OTHER. *All human others.*

The point of this exercise is, once again, to momentarily cut through socially conditioned habitual patterns, specifically, to dissolve the solidity, security, and imprisonment of the "how I look" cave. It is also to dissolve the deep illusion of neutrality and transparency involved in the cultural practice called "seeing oneself." It's easy to look in the mirror and see my habitual, reflected image. It's harder to see that there are limits to our seeing or that, indeed, I can't actually see … me.

I See That I Do Not see

Kimberly: As I strode in front of the mirror, I found it very hard not to try to fix something. I'm used to using the mirror to do my hair, makeup or fix myself up, etc. It was hard to just sit there and not do anything.

I found myself to be very self-critical and self-conscious about how I looked. I realized that I really had never spent even ten minutes in front of a mirror doing nothing but looking at myself, even though I have spent hours getting ready. Then what do we really use a mirror for? Is it an artificial way of covering ourselves and who we really are? It really raised a lot of questions in my mind about how I approach my appearance. I noticed for the first time the lines on my face, the shape of my face, nose, and lips, and the complexity of my eyes and their different colors. We are truly remarkable organisms and yet we can't see our beauty. We spend so much money covering it up—who are we underneath all those products? I definitely will look twice the next time I'm standing in front of a mirror!

In doing this meditation grounded exercise, if we are patient, disciplined, and don't succumb to boredom—if we resist the powerful pull to fall back into the familiar `natural attitude' of the Platonic cave, of media matrix–conditioned common-sense—we can often see a most valuable thing: We can see how much we habitually *don't see.* We can see how much our acquired relationship to the world is one of fundamentally ignoring it. When we stay with the mirror long enough, we tend to cut through our habitual speedy mind. Instead of its merely reflecting back our projections and our familiar confusion laced with mental speed, we begin to perceive more and project less. When we vividly catch that we habitually mistake our thoughts about our self for our self, we come up against a fundamental dimension of Western philosophy in a very personal way: Descartes' famous "I think, therefore I am." We may re-experience this historical Western philosophical preoccupation, however, with a twist in that our habitual mirror portrait is made mostly out of conceptual evaluations and dramatic postures and gestures rather than sense perceptions. Our "I" is mostly composed of thoughts. In that sense, our mirror reflection *reflects* our socialization and our media conditioning rather than our senses.

Scott: Looking in the mirror at myself I saw myself. There was only me in the mirror; I looked the same as I always did. A few minutes later though I began to notice subtle facial characteristics that I hadn't noticed before. My eyebrows are huge! I have the eyelashes of a woman! Pretty soon my whole face looked totally strange to me. I was no longer looking at myself, but a total stranger. This feeling of being apart from myself sporadically appeared every so often in between periods where I saw myself as I did when I first scrutinized myself. Looking back on the experience, I feel that the majority of the time I must be projecting a self-concept of myself when I look at myself instead of my true appearance (somewhat like hearing a tape recording of your voice and noticing that it sounds incredibly unlike what you thought it sounded like). I suppose these unreal images of ourselves reflect the way we wished we looked rather than the way we actually look.

Many of us discovered in this exercise that "I don't look like I thought I looked." This is a discovery, a realization. It is not itself a sensory perception.

Where are we when we are *in* the mirror? Is the reflection in the mirror perhaps another shadow projected on the cave wall? In the magical world of reflections, we are instantly transported into the philosopher's world of epistemological puzzles—puzzles that have haunted Western philosophy for centuries: Is my "self" ultimately reducible to my body? Am I seeing in my reflection what others are seeing when they see me? Does my reflection and, by extension, my world appear identical to me as it does to you? How much is "my world" identical with the world? Is what I am judging *about* what I am seeing, "me," the same or similar to what you, the Other, are judging when you see me? Is beauty in the eyes of the beholder? Is the world in the eyes of the beholder?

Karl: As a prelude to my experiment I decided that it would be useful to picture my face in my mind as well as I could. That way I would not be able to fool myself into thinking that what I saw was what I have always visualized.

I started in on a cursory survey. I examined my face as a single unit, and I was not a bit surprised to find that I resembled myself a great deal. It was when I started to notice the individual units that my features fell apart before my eyes. I began to notice the little scars I have acquired over the years. I never think of them, so I failed to visualize them in my self-imagining. Of course when others see me, they do not fail to see these scars. They are logged away as part of my total appearance. Then all of a sudden my nose looked nothing like I had always seen it. I had always visualized a sharply cut nose, but now it was a roundish sort of nose. I thought I must be letting the experiment get to me so I tried to force the image on the mirror to look like the one in my mind. I looked at it from different angles. I scrunched it around. Finally I tried to simply change the way I saw it in my mind. This was the most successful ploy, but even here I could not hold the image of a sharp nose in my mind for more than a split second. The roundish reality, at least I think it was reality, of my nose kept staring back at me. I started to think about my face as if I were a person I had just met and was seeing for the first time, at which my cheek and jaw line changed. Again rounding out from the sharper images in my self-perception.

As I try and draw conclusions from this experiment, two thoughts are stuck in my mind. It is obvious to me that I am not seen by others as I see me, but another question is whether or not I am perceiving others with my own slant to it. Am I seeing the faces of my fellows or am I just seeing what I lay on top of their features with my own mind?

In deeply engaging in this mirror meditation, we discover that we don't see with our eyes. Generally speaking, every person has eyes that perform the exact same function. If everyone saw with their eyes, we would all see the same things. No, essentially we see with our minds.

Advertising's Eyes: Where Does Advertising End and My Reflection Begin?

Without regard to the actual selling of the product being advertised, without regard to selling anything whatsoever, without regard to money or profit, what do you think advertising *does*? From a cultural historical perspective, we look, talk, and think differently because of advertising. Where does the ad end and the product begin? More pointedly, where does advertising end and my self begin? How much of who we think we are has been infected and infested with advertising culture. How much of who we think we are and who we aspire to be is the dream of this advertising culture? The sociologist C. Wright Mills, in *The Power Elite*, captured the basic social psychological formula of our advertising culture back in its robust, aggressive, and global emergence in the 1950s. The system of advertising has

...not only filtered into our experience of external realities, it has also entered into our very experience of our own selves. They have provided us with new identities and new aspirations of what we should like to be, and what we should like to appear to be ... (1) the media tell us who we are—they give us identity; (2) they tell us what we want to be—they give us aspirations; (3) they tell us how to get that way—they give us technique; and (4) they tell us how to feel that we are that way even when we are not—they give us escape. The gaps between identity and aspiration lead to technique and/or to escape. That is probably the basic psychological formula of the mass media today ... The chief distracting tension of the media is between the wanting and the not having of commodities or of women [and men] held to be good looking.

(Mills 1959:314–315)

After being conditioned by our advertising culture, we no long *see* these products that they are selling but, rather, we see the fulfillment of our dreams *in* these products. Insofar as the medium that advertisers work in is the human mind, advertising is really applied social psychology. As Violet Ray states,

What makes ads so dangerous is that we still want them to come true. Somewhere in our hearts we still believe in the dream life they portray. The issue is not whether ads tell us the truth—they make no pretence to do so. Nor is it that they create illusions or false consciousness for us. None of this gets at their effectiveness in harnessing us to the machinery of consumption. Ads are directed with disarming familiarity at us as individuals, but their effect is to create a social world defined by the products we consume and the expectations they bring with them. What ads are really about is the symbolic VALUE we place on belonging to that society ... In our culture this amounts to a kind of lust for a social world that does not exist anywhere except in the advertisement, and for that reason becomes all the more of an obsession to us.

(Ray 1984:2)

When we see an advertisement, we don't simply see it; rather, we situate ourselves in it: If you buy this product, you will join this world. Our advertising culture has reached such a saturation point that the ad, the image, has now overtaken and superseded the product. You are not paying for the lotion in the container; you are paying for the promise in the advertisement. Though on the conventional surface we are buying the product, on a deeper level we are *buying the advertisement.* The product now *is* the advertisement.

Beauty is displayed and defined within the advertising world, and then a product is offered up as means to obtain it. However, it is also important to understand that no ad stands alone: All ads support all other ads; all ads make reference to all other ads. Whatever the specific *content* that is displayed in any ad, the *form* of advertising itself is always also being displayed. In this sense, *all advertising* also *advertises advertising.* Every time a young beautiful woman is used as a decorative object to promote cars, beer, or vacation spots, she is also selling her image and images of her image. Every time a woman older than 30 is used to promote cleaning products, food, and medicines, it reinforces the prevailing standards of beauty and age and the accompanying values that are transmitted. Frequently in the ad, the 'beautiful advertising person' looks directly at the viewer and creates a "mirror" effect.

> Look in a mirror. If you are a woman, what do you see? The simple mirrors that hang over bureaus and on the backs of closet doors only tell us superficial physical things about ourselves. The real-life mirrors are the media, and for women the most invidious mirror of all is advertising.
>
> (Komisar 1971:304)

The images of advertising viscerally present us with the dominant philosophy of our age, the age of the image, the age of living among the jungle of the surfaces of ever-proliferating mediated representations, the age of advertising.

> *Matthew:* I began to realize that I have been trained to look for my flaws and not to be satisfied with what I have been given...It was at this point that I realized that I was not looking at myself through beginner's eyes. I was looking at myself through advertiser's eyes.

> *Holly:* I began to feel that I was being exposed in front of a panel of judges that were to give some critical rating based on my appearance. I felt exposed to myself and violated by myself. A part of me became one of the judges and was extremely critical of myself. The other half of me

was on the defensive. This side of me knew that I could be a happy and fun person, and that my good qualities would outweigh the bad. But the longer I sat there the larger the critic in me grew. It was as if I could hear the judges in the background laughing at the positive side until it became smaller and smaller. I did not know that I could be so critical of myself. I was truly scared.

A specter is haunting the mirrors of our modern media world, the specter of advertising. That genius of cinema, Frederico Fellini, once said in an interview that each person's face is the perfect expression of the being of that person. How far is that from the established way of seeing ruled by our advertising culture! Instead of seeing our self or someone else for who they are, we see them for what they look like.

The role of advertising, after aggressively establishing a monopoly on our minds, is to clandestinely create a world of mirrors in which people can ongoingly obtain new images of themselves that fit and support the purposes of the overall corporate consumer system. *Who we are and how we look right now is* always inferior *to who we could be and how we could look.* One must grudgingly admire the subtlety with which the advertising media took control of our thoughts and then conditioned us to think that those thoughts were entirely our own. Through this type of mirror function and by its expropriation of our inner experience, advertising tends to make the human into a spectator of his or her own life. Life itself becomes a spectacle. Advertising effectively pulls our feelings up out of ourselves, displays them, and then sells them back to us. Whenever we buy a product, we are at least partially paying for the recovery of our own feelings. We're buying ... "Me." We have thereby turned into creatures who are the commodities we buy.

Why can't we just *simply see* our reflection? Why can't we just accept the way we are? The mirror image is a mere catalyst, a key to set off the psychologically violent, whirring engines of self-criticism, self-hatred, and body-hatred. Our face, our body, are not perfect. In this situation, who is giving the blame? Who is getting the blame? Whose is the critical voice here? Where does this learned, trained, highly shaped criticalness come from? Can we critically use this harsh, negative mirror situation for purposes of liberation? That is can, we turn it around and become critical towards this criticalness itself?

To find this out, we must attain a very still mind, allowing the idea of being perfect to become nonexistent so that there is nothing to compare ourselves with and no need to. If we become very quiet and very still with the mirror and really closely listen, we will hear, like a voice-print recognition machine, the voice of the commercial media and advertising. If we dust this surface of violent, accusatory, and painful judgments, we will find the fingerprints of advertising. "What threatens the body in our time is the temptation to self-loathing induced by those who profit from envy and anxiety in consumers" (Goldstein 1993:5). Schooled through an advertising culture when we look in the mirror, paradoxically we see, above all, *what we are not*. Instead of seeing who we are and what we look like, we see who *they are* (the glamorous, perfect, advertising media models) and what we don't look like. The function of advertising is to create a sense of panic while simultaneously producing and instilling dissatisfaction towards oneself—not an absolute existential dissatisfaction that would *lead to despair or nihilism* but rather a relative, social dissatisfaction toward oneself in comparison to those figures in the advertising world, a dissatisfaction that would *lead to purchasing something*.

Images of perfection bubble up before our eyes as we gaze at ourselves in the mirror. They are an invisible film or shield that comes between us and our reflection. We don't *see*; rather, we *compare* our image. We're conditioned in this advertising culture to confuse seeing with comparing. And where there's comparison, there's competition.

We asked our students, pointedly, to *look* at their reflection, to just look and to see what they could see. When they tried, however, they encountered a strong force that overrode this simple, precise instruction: the force of comparison and judgment, the specter of self-hatred, the hatred of failing to be perfect. Where does this image of perfection come from? Who owns this perfection? Who owns the means of production of perfection and glamour?

From a sociological point of view, 20 minutes in front of the mirror is one of the most ruthless ways of showing us how much our psyches have already been colonized by the commercial advertising media. Analogous to the interiorized self-hatred of minorities for not looking white in a white supremacist society, we have interiorized self-hate in regard to commercial photographic beauty and photographic perfection as presented by the media/advertising industry. Today, as Naomi Wolf says in *The Beauty Myth, How Images of Beauty are used to Oppress Women,* if all the media photos of ethnic minorities in ads were consistently airbrushed and computer-enhanced to always appear a few degrees lighter, whiter, more Caucasian, it would cause a political outrage (1991:82–83). Yet, all the advertising photos are airbrushed and computer-enhanced to create a few degrees more of beauty perfection.

We see, and we say, "My upper lip is too thin, my nose is too wide, my cheeks are too round," and so on. This is very different from seeing and saying, "My upper lip is thin, my nose is wide, my cheeks are round." In comparison to what are my lips *too* thin? Where have we learned to invoke this particular type of judgment? Who or what has been inserted between what we perceive ourselves to be and what we judge ourselves to be? *Too thin* is a reference to a standard—specifically the standard of advertising images we have already intimately ingested and personalized and which now come between ourselves and our reflection in the mirror. We wind up with a completely disfigured idea of ourselves. As one student put it, "I finally see my nose as it is—a mechanism with which to breathe, not a flaw marring my whole character." For a moment, at least, he looked at reality with its own eyes.

Sometimes, when we closely look, we almost literally see how much of an advertisement (especially cosmetic) we have ourselves become.

Ann: My morning ritual has just been completed. Foundation makeup to cover all imperfections in the skin, cornsilk to prevent a shiny face, blush for a natural, healthy look and emphasis or creation of cheekbones, eye shadow for undistinguished eyelids, and mascara for lengthening and thickening of eyelashes have all been applied with various brushes, pencils and sponges. I now stand in front of the mirrored medicine cabinet with my face on. I am now prepared to face the world. It is amazing that all this goop on the outside could make me feel so much more appealing and confident on the inside. It seems sad, but it is true. I wonder for what reason and for whom am I doing all this? I also wonder who taught me that this was the correct thing to do?

Undoubtedly, I am doing it for myself. Everyone likes to look attractive, and attractive has been defined by the media as flawless. Besides, men like attractive women. I would really dislike it if one of my

male friends were to see me without my makeup on. This brings me to
a contradiction which I have not yet resolved. If a man is supposed to
like/love me for what I really am, personality included, then why am I so
obsessed with presenting an image that really is not me? People say that
beauty is only skin deep, but if you look at women in advertisements and
in the media in general, you'd probably think that women were all skin!

We tend to think the attractive photos of ourselves are accurate
reflections. The unattractive photos of ourselves are just bad photos.
We strive, it would seem, to believe that there is a stable, fundamental
way we look, an underlying substance to our ever-changing appearances
that does not change and flicker from moment to moment. In this
regard, however, we are more akin to fire than to earth. Photographs
of ourselves are less like landscape photos than they are similar to
photographs of fire—never the same appearance moment to moment.
We'd like to believe we're more like landscape photographs, that we get
access to ourselves and open up out to others with the stable solidity
of a landscape rather than with the impossible impermanence of a fire.
However, we are flickering all the time to each other. Viewing our self
or viewing another, what is changing is not only what is seen but also
who is looking.

Elissa: I never allow myself to just look at me for no set reason. You
have to be perfect to do that—you have to be worth looking at. And I'm
not the picture perfect image that I wish I was. I kept thinking of the
latest Sports Illustrated magazine—the yearly bathing suit issue. How
do I ever compare with that? Why do I compare myself? It's so hard not
to, when you see photos of people that are so un-real looking. Photos
somehow equal reality in my mind. I believe they are telling the truth
because I never touch-up my own photographs. I automatically assume
that they wouldn't be low down and dirty enough to do it also. I forget
that no one really looks like that. I bet if I saw the latest celebrity model
on the street, I wouldn't recognize her. It seems so ridiculous to me that I
spend so much time to make myself presentable. Every morning I try to
make my outside self come a little closer to the magazine ideal.

Advertising and Beauty Addiction[1]

We are enveloped today by never-ending processions of advertising images. Each day we are bombarded by hundreds and hundreds and hundreds of ads, via newspapers, television, Internet spam, movies, radio, magazines, direct mail, billboards, bumper stickers, clothing logos, poster boards, and so on. The current estimates gauge that we are exposed to about 3,000 distinct ad imprints a day. You would think we'd all be in a state of shell shock. Yet, strangely, this is all very ordinary and familiar. It feels very natural to us. We don't give the ad-vironment a second thought; and furthermore, we don't give the advertisement a second thought. For the most part, we see advertising as trivial, silly, and inconsequential. The prevalent attitude is "Advertising doesn't effect *me*."

We tend to see ourselves as free, autonomous individuals, in complete command of our thoughts and actions. This particular version of freedom and the unique feeling-tone accompanying it is itself largely the result of being "under the influence" of advertising, almost as if advertising were like alcohol or some other drug that put us in a haze or mild stupor. We are in denial of being "under the influence" of advertising. We are conditioned to see ourselves this way and, furthermore, conditioned to see ourselves as unconditioned. As Judith Williamson argues in her classic critique,

> Ads create an "alreadyness" of "facts" about ourselves as individuals: that we are consumers, that we have certain values, that we will freely buy things, consume, on the basis of those values, and so on. We are trapped in the illusion of choice. "Freedom" is in fact part of the most basic ideology, the very sub-structure of advertising. Outside the structure of advertisement themselves, it forms the fundamental argument always used to justify advertising: *that it is part of the freedom of manufactures to compete, and part of our freedom, to choose between the products of that competition.* The idea of freedom is essential to the maintenance of ideology... advertisements work by a process in which we are completely enmeshed... they invite us "freely" to create ourselves in accordance with the way in which they have already created us.
>
> (Williamson 1978:42; emphasis added)

---

1 Some of the following remarks on beauty advertising were first addressed earlier by our colleagues David Boyns and Lorraine McGrane.

Though we may reject individual ads, we don't reject "advertising." In many ways, we are in a state of denial, not toward advertising as such but toward advertisings' real influence and hold us on, personally, individually, and collectively. We deny that we are, in fact, "under the influence." Further, because we do not take the efficacy of advertising seriously, we allow it a dangerous and extremely potent kind of banality. It is through this process of myopia and random, unsolicited absorption of advertising images by which we are subtly coerced and seduced into consumerism. Above all else, advertising is selling buying, or, more precisely, consuming.

Advertisements have become such an ingrained part of our environment that, very simply, we don't really *see* them. Instead, they quietly seep into the background of our consciousness, where their effects on our psyche go unnoticed, unfelt, unsupervised. The ideology of the advertisement lurks within us unexamined and unreflected upon. It is here, in our twilight subconscious, in the stream of our subconscious gossip, where advertising achieves its greatest power over us.

The Hidden Ad

Advertising is a medium that produces and sells images and representations, rather than products. As we all know, on the surface, the purpose of advertising is to coax us into buying products. What we miss, however, is the ad hidden within the ad. For, on a deeper, much more powerful level, the purpose of advertising is to socialize us into becoming a particular type of person, namely a consumer: one whose identity is deeply dependent upon wanting, buying, and possessing consumer products. In the momentary presence of the ad, the consumer becomes dissatisfied not with the way of life of society but with his own life within this society. As the ex-advertising executive, Jerry Mander, says,

> Advertising exists only to purvey what people don't need ... I have never met an advertising person who sincerely believes that there is a need connected to, say, 99 percent of the commodities which fill the airways and the print media ... . Consider the list of the top twenty-five advertisers in the United States. The sell the following products: soaps, detergents, cosmetics, drugs, chemicals, processed foods, tobacco,

alcohol, cars and soda, all of which exist in a realm beyond need. If they were needed they would not be advertised.

(Mander 1978:126–127)

The thrust of advertising manifests itself in the ongoing continuous creation of synthetic needs, desires, and selves. It appeals to illusory "defects" by suggesting that something is wrong with us as we are, that we are somehow inadequate. Hence, advertisings' global effect is to mold us into beings who are perpetually wanting and desiring, craving after the synthetic fancies of the advertising world. *This process turns identity and the search for individuality essentially into a shopping experience.* Its intent is to shape us into human beings whose fundamental quality is *to be constantly preoccupied with wanting something we don't have.* In effect, advertising shapes us to be the type of human being that is most useful to the profit-driven, privately organized economy. To keep consumption healthy, and therefore keep the economy under corporate capitalism healthy, advertisers manipulate, magnify, and fabricate our needs. Advertisers accomplish this by psychologically inflating commodities with symbols, dreams, and images. The objective of the advertisement, then, is not so much to sell us products but, more, to seduce us into a hallucinatory world of artificially generated imagery, to draw us into the world of the advertisement, to create and continuously re-create ourselves as consumers. In this process, advertising fosters and reinforces a peculiar kind of self-hatred: not a wild, amorphous self-hatred but a self-hatred that seeks to tranquilize itself in buying consumer products.

It is in this region wherein the awesome and terrifying power of the ad lies, dormant and unexamined. What is being sold along with products is beauty, prestige, love, friendship, sexual intimacy, status, wealth, desirability, youth, social acceptance, femininity, masculinity, power, happiness, popularity, glamour, success, romance, sex appeal, and independence. Thus, the commodities solicited by the advertisements "become not ends in themselves but overvalued means for acquiring acceptable ends" (Schudson 1984:7). Moreover, these acceptable ends or qualities then become deeply and forcefully *commodity-dependent*. A displacement occurs whereby:

- Personal and social qualities are now seen and defined as *emanating* from possessions;

- These qualities are *only* achieved and manifested through commodities; and
- These possessions as commodities are *purchasable.*

Hence, beauty, femininity, and glamour are not only possessions for sale but are defined and recognized only through products. According to the brilliant, renegade advertiser, Howard Gossage, this remarkable power of advertising can be seen as a sort of modern-day magic, going beyond reason into a magical realm where "the product is its advertising." In this sense, we are bewitched by advertising magic.

Beauty for Sale

Selling beauty has become a multi-billion dollar business. Beauty itself is now a commodity—a commodity defined, contained, and imprisoned by an advertising culture. "The beauty myth tells a story: The quality called 'beauty' objectively exists. Women must want to embody it and men must want to possess women who embody it" (Wolf 1991:120). The cover girl of today represents the ideal in feminine beauty, an ideal that is intricately tailored and bound to advertisers who must create needs and markets for products to generate profits, both for themselves and their corporate clients. Women spend billions of dollars each year on makeup, skin products, nail polishes, body hair removers, perfumes, personal hygiene products, lingerie, clothes, weight-reducing products, and plastic surgery. Along with these commodities, they buy the images ... they buy the dreams ... they buy the values ... they buy the advertisements ... and most of all, *they become the advertisements.*

There is, of course, nothing inherently wrong with wanting to look attractive, sexy, or feminine. It must be understood that this is *not* an anti-beauty argument. The concern, rather, is with the images, values, and dreams that are *being sold* to us and changing our views of ourselves and of our beauty, those media practices and media products that literally depend upon making us perpetually neurotic and uncomfortable about who we are.

Our hope is to energize you to become more aware of the effect living inside of the media matrix has on us all. As Jean Kilbourne, the creator of "Killing Us Softly," argues,

By remaining unaware of the profound seriousness of the ubiquitous influence, the redundant message, the subliminal impact of advertisements, we ignore one of the most powerful "educational" forces in this culture, one that greatly affects our self-images, our ability to relate to each other, and our concepts of success and worth, love and sexuality, popularity and normalcy

(Kilbourne 1977:293).

We are so enveloped by these images that it has become very difficult to distinguish between our own *self-generated* conceptions and beliefs about who we are and those conceptions and beliefs generated by the advertising world that have somehow infiltrated us, sort of "sleeper cells" in our own psyche.

We think it vital and valuable to raise and practice critical self-questioning in pursuit of media therapy and societal change, hence our repeated experimental use of sociological "koans" to yank us "off-program." How much of who I think I am has been infested with advertising culture? How much of who I think I am and who I aspire to be is the dream of this corporate advertising culture?

As with television, we are so used to thinking of advertisement as *mere advertisements*. It's not until we pull away the hazy, dreamlike gauze of semi-hypnotic attentiveness that comes over us in the presence of ads that we can attempt to see their real force, energy, and intent. When you re-experience these dreamy advertisements in the broad daylight of critical consciousness, they no longer have their everyday status of ordinariness or acceptability. Ads in their ordinary context of advertising have the status of Dr. Jeykell. Stripped of that context and made to stand in the light of the day, they reveal themselves more as Mr. Hyde. What had been innocent, neutral, and ordinary, socially and politically acceptable, suddenly stands out as monstrous and distorted, as genuinely and deeply revolting.

Beauty and the Beast

Unquestionably, one of the grossest injustices played out upon us, particularly women, has been by the beauty industry and its advertising. The beauty industry and its world of beauty fetishism has done more than any other socially sanctioned institution to glorify the sardonic world of Ambrose Bierce, and to contribute to the definition of women as, before all else, spectacles and appearance-objects. In Bierce's world,

> To men a man is but a mind. Who cares what face he carries or what form he wears? But woman's body is the woman... A woman absent is a woman dead.
>
> (Bierce 1911:9)

For a woman, Bierce's world implies, what is essential is not who you are but more importantly what you look like. You *are* your appearances. The cover *is* the book. It is a complete domination of style over substance. Bierce's world is the world that has been created by the beauty industry through advertising. The images of women that we see in advertisements are simply those of ornamentally embellished mannequins, whose sole existence seems to pivot upon the obsessive maintenance of their comely image amid the turbulent abuses of everyday life.

It is precisely this kind of psychological turmoil that the beauty industry thrives on. By generating self-doubt and discontent, advertisements entice a woman to consume synthetic beauty. They function to encourage women not only to see aspects of themselves within the advertisement but to see aspects of the advertisement within themselves. A woman is thus trained to become obsessively self-scrutinizing. The spectacle within the ad always depicts a future self, a self that you need to be to achieve the necessary and proper sense of self-esteem.

Advertisements work because they are able to subtly persuade a woman *that there is always something wrong with her.* There is always something presently wrong with her, or something about to be, soon to be, wrong with her. The ads act as a corrosive acid on her self-esteem. They appropriate a woman's sense of self-worth and replace it with a vicarious, synthetic self, a cosmetic self that is consumed by, and in turn consumes her.

Artificial Reality

If men define situations as real, they are real in their consequences...

(W. I. Thomas 1928:572)

Advertising presents a perfect world—that is just a few dollars away. These ideal images of beauty by which women are compared, both by themselves and by others, are presented in advertising as being very real and attainable through the use of products. However, the truth is that they are quite non-real, illusory, and non-attainable. They exist nowhere except inside the advertisement itself. Nobody in the real world outside of the advertisement looks like, or even *can* look like the ideal image within the ad, including the models. The images of these flawless women are manufactured through the use of professional hair stylists, makeup artistic, hi-tech cameras, special lighting, digital airbrushing, and sophisticated computers that can literally compose photographic images. (See the *Dove Campaign* on YouTube.) Imperfections are *technically masked*, whereas perfection is *technically created*. Hours and hours are spent creating that one picture-perfect image. The models are different, but they all adhere to the same narrowly defined look. And because these perfect picture images proliferate throughout our ad-vironment, we become vulnerable to their illusions and quite susceptible to seeing them as very real and genuine. The real-life models themselves have often been physically altered through plastic surgery and cosmetic dental work. These women weren't all born with perfect (as defined by the beauty industry) noses, cheekbones, smiles, and breasts. Even the full lips that are sporadically "in" have in many cases simply been purchased. These women are not perfect from head to toe. In fact, model images are sometimes dismembered, and the final image, while appearing to belong to one person both visually and logically, is actually the composite of more than one model. There are even some models, called "part models," who are only used for a specific, highly photogenic part of their body such as their hand, legs, feet, or buttocks. Even very beautiful women in the media have had their hands doubled by a hand model in advertisements. The same parts are often used repeatedly, so a person could be looking at two or more ads featuring the faces of different models but all baring the exact same hands that belong to someone else. This holds true for other parts of their body as well.

These models are made, not born. Consequently, both the models and the images we see are creations: photographic pieces of commercial "art." These perfect images are manufactured through layers and layers of hidden artificiality. Left to their own, these women could *never* capture their own photographic images. Yet, to a large degree, *we believe these images are real*. Most people are completely unaware of the degree to which these photographs are artificially fabricated—or, if they are aware, they cannot bring that awareness vividly enough to mind in the seeing-is-emotionally-believing, captivating presence of the ad. Trained by the advertising culture, we internalize these images and compare ourselves very personally to a mythical ideal. We become lost in a world of mirrors where illusions and shadows on the cave wall become more real that reality itself.

We are creatures of caricature caught, entranced, and mesmerized by an advertising culture. Our advertising culture sells us synthetic selves and an enchanted world in which these synthetic selves are the inhabitants. Advertising creates for us an artificial reality, a pseudo-world in which all experiences are indirectly media-ated by representations and images of experience. Because of its success and influence, we have a tendency to suppress and reduce the actual, real, direct experience of our lives, of our lived existential selves. We redirect our energies and live vicariously through media spectacles. The Muses behind advertising are the creators of a fantasy world and, as we unconsciously portray and perform the role of consumer, we literally buy into this pseudo-reality and support its misgivings. In the vast, global, Platonic cave, the shadows before us are now indeed more magnetically seductive and colorful than any "reality" could ever be. Thomas de Zengotita (2006) relates in *Mediated*, as we mentioned before, that one of his techie friends responded to him upon reading his criticism of the flattering, delusional unreality of this mediated reality, "What's so great about reality?"

Eating Disorders

The critical way we tend to view ourselves when we do something as simple as looking into the mirror has more consequences than a non-flattering comparison to people we see in the media. Eating disorders have become so common that, when we now ask our classes whether they know someone with an eating disorder, almost all hands go up. According to the American Medical Association, eating disorders rank as the third most common major illness of teenage girls, with 5 to 10 million sufferers. One million men and boys also have eating disorders.

The assault of the media on our body image is relentless and lifelong and has staggering results. The bombardment of images of thin beautiful people has helped create a multi-billion dollar dieting industry and masses of individuals unhappy with their own bodies. Forty percent of 9–10-year-olds are even trying to lose weight, and 81 percent have said they have tried dieting at this young age. By the time these kids reach high school, 63 percent of the girls and 16 percent of the guys will be on diets at any one time. A Stanford University study found that 68 percent of students felt worse about their body image after reading women's magazines for a short period. Young girls in one survey even reported being afraid of becoming fat more than nuclear war, cancer, or losing their parents. Being afraid of becoming fat compared to the other options seems preposterous at first glance but, in a media-saturated culture that glorifies these images, becoming fat is more "real" to most teen girls in comparison to the other situations that are seemingly hypothetical.

What is even more frightening is this obsession to be thin is based on an unrealistic image of beauty created by the media. Jean Kilbourne has done much to point out the portrayal of the image of women in the media and the negative effects on our perceptions in her lectures, books, and films. She has documented that the standard of beauty in the media is not "real" or even obtainable. Now computers are even creating completely animated models so no touch-ups are needed. (Consequently, neither are people.) Shockingly, the average model is now 23 percent under normal body weight, down sharply from 8 percent 20 years ago. It is not surprising in this bombardment of "unreal" images that women feel dissatisfied with their appearance. Many young women are at war with their bodies and literally dying to be thin. The following long passage is from one of our former students, a young woman who has personally fought this battle. Her story is powerful and something that many of us might relate to. It is a vivid example of the consequences of the medias' distortion of our perceptions of our bodies and of the importance of accepting who we are. There are, of course, *many* causal factors at work in the etiology of a severe clinical eating disorder. Our intention in including Kristin's report here is more to underscore the pervasive, normative media imagery that interweaves her story.

Kristin: I was 12 years old the first time I made myself throw up. It was the day we watched the movie in health class about the very subject, bulimia. I went home and ate my usual half a container of Ben and Jerry's Coffee Heath Bar Crunch, but then I ate the other half, and half a box of Wheat Thins and anything else I could possibly get my hands on. Then I went upstairs to the bathroom, took my toothbrush, sat down before the toilet, and my struggle began.

I had been skinny my whole life and I could eat anything I wanted. But as I started to grow into a young woman, all I could think about were the constant comments everyone around me was making. "You're so lucky now but just wait till you get older, all that food is going to catch up with you." "Enjoy being so skinny now, it won't last forever." "Just wait until you start developing ..." That was who I was, the skinny one. But I had become so afraid of what was going to happen to me, I was determined to put a stop to it before it could even start, before I could gain a pound.

Throughout high school, things got better, then worse when I discovered that anorexia was even better than bulimia, then slightly better, then so much worse. I finally ended up just flip-flopping between the two approaches all while challenging myself to eat as little as possible while exercising as much as I could. Going in and out of hospitals, seeing more therapists, psychiatrists, psychologists, doctors, and nutritionists, than I could count was the next stage in this cycle. My parents and friends were all angry with me for doing this to myself, telling me that I just wanted attention and how ashamed they were of me. But no one ever wanted to just listen to me and understand. Couldn't they see I just wanted to look good? It is so much easier to judge and get angry I thought. Even through all of this I didn't think I had a problem.

Then I went off to college happy and ready to be healthy and make a fresh start. My first visit home, I had apparently put on the "freshman 15" because everyone I saw told me how much weight I had gained and how great I looked. Unfortunately, I only heard the part about how much weight I had gained.

Then I started my sophomore year of college. My best friend Nicole and I were so much alike. We were the same height, super skinny (at least in everyone else's eyes) and could not get enough of fashion magazines. We spent hours, days, months, combing through Vogue, W, Elle, anything we could fine, in awe of all the "heroin chic" models. We meticulously cut out the fashion pages and ads and hung them on our walls. The walls all around my desk and bed were plastered with pictures of these incredibly beautiful women with impossibly perfect bodies. We weren't attracted to the women; we were obsessed with wanting to be these women. Those pictures were there to remind me everyday what I wanted to be, what I was working so hard for. I wanted to be them; I wanted their unachievable, airbrushed, flawless bodies. Every night these images were the last thing I saw before I went to sleep and the first thing I saw when I awoke every morning. Not to mention every TV show and movie I saw also validated my obsession. Yet I would stand in the mirror and obsess about my thighs being too flabby or having cellulite. "I want stick thighs like models have" is what we would say. And that's what I would think of as I spent 30 minutes on the Stairmaster and 30 minutes on the bike after eating a bowl of fat free cereal with fat free milk that I then purged right back up. But yet, I still saw nothing wrong with myself. I thought I was just a college girl trying to keep in shape, trying to be healthy, trying to lose the "freshman 15."

That November I went home for Thanksgiving break. My ex-boyfriend and another high school friend of mine stopped by my parent's house to see me. The look on their faces as I walked into the living room was that of utter shock and sadness. Each hugged me so tightly yet so tenderly as if afraid to break me. I knew I had lost weight, but their reactions were haunting. As we sat and chatted that look of sympathy, as if I were dying, remained on their faces and the visit was uncomfortable, not really knowing what to talk about without talking about my weight. My ex tried to pull me aside and talk to me, saying how worried he was about me, that I was way too skinny but I didn't want to listen, I didn't want to believe him.

The next day I could not get my ex's face out of my head. He had never looked at me that way before, just unbearably sad for me, afraid for me. I convinced myself that they were just over reacting. I looked good. I got out of the shower and decided to finally weigh myself. I had come to loathe the scale and avoided it at all costs. All through high school I had a love hate relationship with it. I would weigh myself everyday and then hide from it, afraid of what it would say. I remember reading that when dieting you should avoid weighing yourself and focus more on how you feel and how your clothes fit, so that's what I obsessed about, seeing what clothes I could still fit in, seeing how small a size I could buy. Everyone I knew commented on my weight, constantly asking me how much I weighed. My friends would all ask how much weight I lost, the guys joked about how far they could throw me, the girls who I felt were angry and bitter that I was getting all the attention telling me I was too skinny and that there was no way I weighed 100 pounds. I knew I had lost weight but I was so scared to prove them right, to admit that I had a real problem. But my ex had no motive, he was being honest, maybe I did loose a few more pounds than I thought; but I looked good and they were wrong.

Sopping wet, in a towel, I stood on the scale. As I look down tears streamed down my face and I just stood there, feet glued to the scale, unable to comprehend what I saw. I was 5'7" and I weighed 83 pounds. 83 pounds! 83 pounds is what I weighed when I was 12!

I finally could admit I needed help but I didn't know how to get help or where to turn. But then someone came into my life able to give me what I had needed all along, I found someone who believed in me, someone who listened to me without being judged. Someone I could talk to when I slipped who didn't get angry with me. It didn't happen in a day, a week, a month or year. Looking back I realize now that this has been the hardest thing that I have ever had to deal with. It took 5 years for me to get control of "it" rather than having "it" control me. And it took another 4–5 years to understand what it truly meant to love myself and to be happy with who I am. And just like an alcoholic, I will always take things each day at a time; I will always be recovering from eating disorders. When I feel myself slipping, thinking I am fat, feeling sick from eating too much, I have places inside of me I can go, I have people that care about me to whom I can turn. It will never go away, but it no longer controls me. I may always be able to pick out silly flaws with my body, but I have learned to embrace my body and cherish my body. I find ways of exercising that are fun. All things in moderation. You can enjoy food and not hate yourself in the morning. There are so many more things in life to focus on; food and my body image are now at the bottom of the list. I'm not going to lie, they will always be on my list, but I won't ever let them creep up to the top.

Naked/Nude: Another Round of Warfare with the Looking Glass

Most of us have been deeply socialized into not observing our naked bodies. We are trained to not look certain places, then to not think certain places. In one version of the biblical tradition, by the might of God and the fault of Adam and Eve, we have all been given a life sentence to wear clothing. We almost never do anything naked other than take showers. We always need something to cover our bodies, whether home alone or outside in the public world. Wearing clothes has become "natural" and not wearing clothes "unnatural."

In his book and video, *Ways of Seeing*, John Berger offers a provocative analysis of how the ways of seeing embodied, taught, and transmitted by the tradition of Western European oil painting continue today in the conventions of commercial advertising. The perspectives, values, and gender relations of "The Nude" in this painting tradition are especially relevant for images of women (and therefore also for men) in advertising. Berger offers the following characterization:

> To be naked is to be oneself. To be nude is to be seen by others and not recognized for oneself. A naked body has to be seen as an object in order to become nude. Nakedness reveals itself. Nudity is placed on display. To be naked is to be without disguise. To be on display is to have the surface of one's own skin … turned into a disguise which… can never be discarded. The nude is condemned to never being naked. Nudity is a form of dress. In the average European oil painting of the nude the principal protagonist is never painted. *He is the spectator* in front of the picture and he is presumed to be a man. Everything is addressed to him…But he, by definition, is a stranger … with his clothes on.
>
> (Berger 1972:54; emphasis mine)

To be naked is natural, an existential presence. Under our clothes, as it were, we are all naked. To be nude, on the other hand, is a purely visual, aesthetic presence. Being nude means that there is an awareness of being seen. When you are alone you are naked; when you are in a magazine, you are nude. In this part of the Looking-Glass self experiment, we personally "tried on" Berger's way of seeing in reference to our own bodies.

> *Lorraine:* I live with my boyfriend. The only time I'm ever really naked is when he's not there … otherwise I'm always nude, no matter how naturally naked I can manage to look.

Women's Mirror: The Jury Behind the Glass

> To men a man is
> but a mind. Who cares
> What face he carries or
> what form he wears?
> But woman's body is the woman
>
> (Ambrose Bierce 1911:9)

> The condensation and freezing of female be-ing is nothing new … a woman preoccupied who obsessively examines herself in a mirror, … is looking through male lenses.
>
> (Daly 1978:232–233)

First, we look at how the women experienced this experiment; then the men.

The women in our classes did, overall, have a more tortuous time engaging in this experiment. Their sexual value appearance was LOUD, often overwhelming. As one remarked, "The mirror experiment revealed to me a self-hate that I try to cover with superficial self-confidence. This experiment truly hurt my feelings."

Within the triad of the mirror, the body, and advertising, there has evolved a profoundly deep relation of inter-destruction, like a bad marriage gone pathological, demonic.

> *Lisa:* At first I was totally repulsed and my first, second, and third impulse was to put my clothes back on and save myself from this misery. But I decided to stick it out. Although I admittedly do not have the perfect body, it's an OK one and more importantly, it's the only body I've got. So I decided that it would be OK to like myself anyway, in spite of

my hips. The difficult part came when I tried to see myself nude. After observing myself naked I thought I would have this next part wired, boy was I wrong. It took a couple of minutes to imagine myself as nude for the viewing or observation of someone other than myself. I never imagined that I'd feel so self conscious. Suddenly, my body was not right and I felt extremely uncomfortable. I know that when I am alone, I can deal with my imperfections or at least ignore them, but God help me if I ever have to take my clothes off in front of anyone else. I become this modest, shy, frightened thing that has to either go into a private changing room or hide behind the nearest large piece of furniture. I ended this experiment a tad early but it still made me ask some pretty serious questions of myself. The most frightening of these questions is can I define where I begin and advertising or media end, and my answer to that is that I have no idea. My view of myself and what I should look like is so confused with what the model and the latest Lancome ad is. I am not sure of where I learned to look at myself this way but I think that it has something to do with the amount of television that I watched as a young child. I feel as though I have so internalized the standards of the advertising world that I will never be able to look at myself with any degree of reality.

Terri: Being "nude" was a much more familiar experience. Certainly not more comfortable, only more familiar. I am "nude" whenever I put on makeup, mugging in the mirror to see how the makeup will look with various expressions underneath it. I am "nude" when the construction workers greet me so loudly. I am "nude" when I know someone is watching me, causing me to walk in a funny, stilted manner. Posing. I felt, while looking in the mirror, that my face, and its expressions, were more involved in making me "nude" than any part of my body. Being "nude" is giving, perhaps not so willingly, a part of oneself to an observer. Their opinion is what matters.

Something more than our ancient and all-too-human anxiety about non-perfection is going on here. What is the source of the pain that we witness so poignantly in these naked/nude exercises? Where does the mirror image end and my self begin? Where does advertising end and my self begin? We have all been socialized into having an ongoing, heightened preoccupation with how-we-look-to-others. The ad industry generates a specific kind of social psychology, an induced self-hate together with an inflated self-preoccupation. As consumers, we become egomaniacs with deep inferiority complexes.

The formula operating here seems to be: we do not look like the media advertisements, *therefore* we are ugly. Or, we look like the media advertisements, *therefore* we are attractive.

Men's Mirror

> Men are exposed to male fashion models but do not see them as *role* models.
>
> (Wolf 1991: 57)

Scott: The first thing I noticed when I looked at myself in the mirror was that this didn't seem all that unusual—for some reason I had thought it would. I had thought that, having hardly ever really looked at my own body, and never been without clothes except to take a shower or sleep, it would be strange and embarrassing. But I wasn't self-conscious at all; in fact I was interested.

I began to see that there were in fact many different ways of looking at myself. One way was to be self-conscious about being seen naked, even though I was the only person seeing. This way paid attention to my slouch, the thinness of my arms and chest, my slightly bow-legged knees. I was concerned with the fact that I will never be terribly good-looking, and this seemed to be an excuse for covering up my body with clothes and acting as normal as possible in hopes that people wouldn't notice that I wasn't very good looking. This point of view also noticed that the face and genitals were the two centers of attention on the naked body, and that by hiding the genitals I was putting everything into my face, which wasn't so great either. In short, it was a way of evaluating my body in terms of how I thought other people would judge it.

Another point of view that I had was a strong identification with my body as a part of myself. This is what made the experience interesting and even enjoyable in a way. It was almost like a reunion, a reinforcement of the ego with the body, basically narcissism. There was nothing sexual or egotistical about this, just a lack of shame and a little perplexity at why shame would be there in the first place. I had the idea that there was no good reason why people should not walk around naked all the time. This seemed somehow cliché, but there still seemed to be an element of truth in it.

There were two other ways of seeing my body that were less pronounced. For brief moments I would see it as just a thing, without any judgment about whether it was good or bad or any attachment to it. This was difficult to do on purpose; it just seemed to happen as a result of my lack of familiarity with my own body and resulting inability to place what I was seeing into a consistent framework. The other way of seeing was myself as a man, in terms of gender. This did not seem strong at all, which bothered me a bit since it seemed to be a part of the assignment. But it just wasn't there and I was tempted to chalk it up to a superior ability to see myself outside of a gender framework. There was a lack of sexuality about the experience that was almost a relief. But then a funny thing happened: I put my clothes back on and became a man again. There was something about the ritual of putting clothes on that was like stepping into a role, a gender identity…It was more like I was dressing myself in the idea of manhood, and even though I don't consider myself terribly masculine, the idea was powerful…It was a return to being normal and the idea of being a man was very much a part of being normal--much more than I had thought. I began to care once again about how I would look to other people … . It seemed that this simple, innocent act of wrapping cloth around ourselves to prevent self-consciousness and the stares of others had, in some ways, the opposite effect.

I Cannot See Me

Self-consciousness exists in itself and for itself only insofar as it exists in and for another self-consciousness; that is, it exists only by being recognized and acknowledged.

(Hegel, *Phenomenology of Spirit*. Debord cpt 9)

The Other teaches me who I am .

(Sartre 1966:366)

How can an individual get outside himself (experientially) in such a way as to become an object to himself? This is the essential psychological problem of selfhood or of self-consciousness…The individual experiences himself as such, not directly, but only indirectly, from the particular standpoints of other individual members of the same social group, or from the generalized standpoint of the social group as a whole to which he belongs. For he enters his own experience as a self or individual, not directly or immediately, not by becoming a subject to himself, but only in so far as he first becomes an object to himself just as other individuals are objects to him … and he becomes an object to himself only by taking the attitudes of other individuals toward himself within a social environment.

(Mead 1962:138)

I see you and you see me. I don't see me, and you don't see you. Like a mirror, we register and reflect the other in front of us. Further, like a mirror we can't reflect our self. Each of us is sort of in the situation of the invisible man. We can see all others but not our self. *Why do we want to see our self?* Why do we want to know, or rather, why do we want to *experience*, what others see when they look at us? How and why have we been socially conditioned and encouraged to zero in less on the substantive, pulsating, living reality of others we encounter and more on the shadowy reflection of how others are seeing … us, how others are judging … us?

Charles Horton Cooley, a famous American sociologist living at the beginning of the twentieth century, developed the term *looking-glass self*. He held that the growth of the self stems from social interaction rather than biological instincts—there is no innate, natural sense of self and self-identity. The machinery by which this self is produced he saw as threefold: (1) Imagining our own appearance to the other person (2) imagining her or his judgment on that appearance (3) experiencing some sort of self-feeling of pride or shame, favorable or unfavorable, regarding that appearance and judgment. Though we may misjudge the way others see us, we still always use this method to learn our appearance and our identity. From this sociological perspective, there really can be no self without interaction. There can be no self without society.

Some Theoretical Remarks on the Discipline of Sociology

Sociology studies the collective forces that work upon us, and it studies the way we project reality, the ways we collude and participate in constructing reality. We are totally and completely social beings, which is to say, "We" is fundamental, "I" is derivative. We inter-are. That is, we believe, one of the fundamental contributions of sociology to our conversations about the human condition.

In terms of intellectual history, sociology dissolves and deconstructs Descartes foundation of "I think, therefore I am." It addresses that which precedes and underlies "I" or "ego." It is true that "I" live my life. "I" share about my experience. "I" share my life with others, and/or "I" isolate myself from others. Yet, nevertheless, from a sociological perspective, prior to all that "I" is "We"—prior to my speech is our language. The words I am expressing at this very moment or that you are reading at this very moment *are not mine* nor *are they yours*. The nature of words, of language, of speech and communication is intimately intertwined with the nature of collective society, of "we," of our culture. The sociological vision focuses, as it were, on that which exists in the spaces through which we move. The focus is not "I" as the subject who is moving, nor the objects "I" move toward or away from. The focus is the in-between, it is that which comes between "I" and other. If society vanished, "I" would cease to exist.

Insofar as I am human, I am not isolated. I am always already in relationship. If I feel fundamental aloneness or loneliness, it is always already in relationship to others who I am not connecting to. To experience aloneness, it is necessary to be in relationship to others whom I am experiencing my aloneness next to. My relationship to others (what Heidegger calls my being-with-others) is the necessary context and horizon upon which I experience my aloneness, my loneliness, my isolation—or even my solitude (to use a positive image). This relates very directly to George Herbert Mead's analysis of language and our *social* nature in *Mind, Self, And Society*. After the accomplishment of interiorizing society and language, I am forever after *with* others, I am forever after *in* relationship, deeply immersed in some form of interior conversation. For Mead, it is only after this human biological organism interiorizes social relationship that "I" emerges. Thus, "I" is, at bottom, *compressed relationship*. Mead holds that society precedes the self. Social relationship composes my self. "I" am not "I" as an isolated monad but as an upsurge of relationship. "We" precedes and composes "I."

If I am transported to a desert island or a remote planet and have no contact with any other human being for the rest of my life, nevertheless, I am not alone, which is to say I am not alone in an absolute sense. Being alone in an absolute sense is thus impossible or only possible prior to socialization, prior to interiorizing language and society. I will be talking to my self forever after—which is to say I will be in conversation with the generalized Other. I may have no immediate, concrete contact with an actual other, but I will never be without the imagined Other, the remembered Other, and the unconscious, structural-self-Other that allows and makes possible the experience of "myself." Aloneness in an absolute sense would be when the Other vanishes totally—which would be simultaneously the disappearance of "my self." The very possibility of being-alone requires that Other; it requires the noticed absence of the presence of the Other.

> *Sandra:* While I was looking at myself for the experiment I really saw myself. Usually I see myself through others' eyes. I think about what others see, not what I see…I came to the conclusion that I've never really been that concerned about what I look like for myself, only for what others see.

> *Clarissa:* I felt a yearning to have the experience of encountering myself as others did. I wanted to grab a hold of myself and look straight into my own eyes as though it were possible for there to be two of me at once.

Cooley's sociological approach toward the self was greatly deepened and expanded by George Herbert Mead. Charles Morris addressed this aspect in his introduction to Mead's work:

> Instead of beginning with individual minds and working out to society, Mead starts with an objective social process and works inward through the importation of the social process….into the individual….The individual has then taken the social act into himself. Mind remains social; even in the inner forum so developed thought goes on by one's assuming the roles of others and controlling one's behavior in terms of

such role taking....The person here has not merely assumed the role of a specific other, but of any other participating in the common activity; he has generalized the attitude of role-taking. In one of Mead's most fertile concepts he has taken the attitude or role of the generalized other. The generalized other....may be regarded as the universalization of the process of role-taking.

(Mead 1962: xxii–xxviii)

We would like to see our self *as* others see us. We would like to "take the role of the other" (in Mead's sense and also in Sartre's) and *actually* see our self. On a basic level, this is what we conventionally believe we are doing when we look at ourselves in the mirror: I am momentarily able to be literally transported outside myself, turn around, and look at myself and experience exactly what another person sees when they look at me. When, however, we closely, precisely, and simply observe our reflection in the mirror for 20 minutes, this apparently self-evident, obvious state of affairs begins to dissolve. An existentially unsettling question arises: Can I see myself? Can I actually see my face? It would seem that our appearance is never directly available to us—only to others.

The point is not "to see oneself" but "to see oneself as one is seen by the Other." To elucidate this phenomenon more precisely, we shift over into first-person, "I" language: I want to know what it is when you see me. It's not a question of how I appear but of how I appear to you. How I appear in your world, through your eyes, in your mind. This is the impossible dream and the impossible feat. I want to see myself without looking at a mirror; or rather I want to see myself *without looking through my eyes, through my mind*. If there really were a magic mirror, I would look in it and *I* wouldn't see *my* reflection but rather *I* would see what *you see* when you look at me. I wouldn't be seeing myself, actively, as it were. I would be magically projected into the consciousness of the Other, I would be somehow magically injected into *you* and then I would be *on the other side*, as it were. Then I could look at the world through your eyes and through your mind—but I wouldn't actually be interested in looking at the world but rather at one particular person in the world, namely *me*. To repeat, the point is not "to see oneself" but rather "to see oneself *as one is seen* by the Other." I will somehow get at the truth of how I am for you only by momentarily *being you*.

I want to see myself through your eyes, through your mind. I need to be you for a moment so that I can look at me. I know and I am haunted by the fact that I am different for you than I am for me. I am other than I am for myself for you. I seek to bridge that insurmountable gap, that chasm, by momentarily being you. It will not do for me to imagine what you see when you see me, when you think me, because then all I am getting is an extension of me. My imagination is an extension of me and hence doesn't really give me access to that which is completely *your* experience of me—completely free of contamination of me and by me.

> *Gina:* These exercises brought to mind some thoughts I've had in the past. Several years ago I was struck by the realization that I have a face but I'll never really see it. The impact of this was actually somewhat frightening. I will never really know what I look like. My image changes even from mirror to mirror, altered by imperfections and wavy areas in the glass. We seem to constantly seek a reflection of ourselves in other people and it's disconcerting that this reflection changes from person to person. Why do some people find me pretty while others find me plain? What do I truly look like? Why do I identify myself with a face that I can't even see?
>
> I am amazed at what a narcissistic being I am. I can't even look at another person without being more intrigued with what he or she sees in me. And how easily my self image is shaken and distorted by how I think I am viewed by others. This experiment has been an enlightening one.

Every time we step in front of the mirror, we momentarily catch, at the speed of perceptual light, a new and strange reflection, and then, with the speed of thought, we see it as *my* reflection.

> *James:* After about five minutes I looked different. My face began to lose some of its distinctiveness. I saw not so much my face, but just a face. This was not easy to grasp, for like most of us I have become very attached to my face. I am used to thinking of it as mine. It seems that when I look at an image of myself in a mirror it is I that gives the image its personhood, its display of self. For without me observing the image, the mirror is nothing more than a piece of glass.

As Sartre stresses in *Being and Nothingness*, my being-for-others, my outside, as it were, is never directly accessible to me. I experience you and you experience me, but I can never experience your experience of me and, likewise, you can never experience my experience of you. I sense that I am an object for others, but what that object is I can never directly, immediately apprehend. What that experience of me is, I can never directly experience. The structure of this world of intersubjectivity is both quite precarious and perpetually vulnerable. It produces a kind of subtle pheromone of ongoing interactional anxiousness when we are directly in the presence of each other—precisely because I can never see me as you see me. And yet....and yet....I am haunted by wanting to accomplish this impossible feat.

There is a radical and profoundly existential democracy built into the very fact of socially sharing a world with others. We are democratically naked, exposed one to the other. We always have been. Paradoxically, because we sense this, therefore we each try in interaction to get control of this situation. We try, as Goffman says, to manage the impression we give off to others and thereby attempt to gain some control over what they are thinking about us.

And *what* are we trying to control? We try to gain control over their freedom. We do all this, of course, in vain for, as Sartre insists, they are always and forever free to make of us what they will....as we are of them. Once this in-vain realization becomes deep enough and real enough, we are to some degree finally *free from control*. That is to say, we are free from the world of thought control and impression management, free from endlessly trying to control the thoughts that others have of us, and perhaps even free from our own thoughts of ourselves, free from over-identifying with thoughts and evaluations altogether.

In terms of a Buddhist psychology, another aspect is also at work here. When we fixate on that which seems solid and continuous, our mind tricks itself into thinking it, too, is solid and continuous. The sense of continuity and self-sameness gives us the illusion that there is some ongoing, continuous witness, some permanence. This ultimate "I" is an assumption and never really perceived nor experienced. When we examine our experience of the mirror carefully, minutely, we never discover a solid, continuous self.

The Looking Glass Other—Close Encounters of the Third Kind

> *Sarah:* I sit next to people all the time in class. I can't believe that by
> rotating my gaze by 90 degrees (from the teacher to the person next to
> me), that my energy would skyrocket, my heart would start pounding,
> and I would feel a strong desire to release my nervous tension through
> laughter or talking. It was like I just broke the law. These are symptoms
> of a shoplifter, not of a person sitting in class! It is amazing to not only
> realize the mental strain we experience by breaking these unwritten rules
> but also the apparent physical strain!

How many people do you know who really look at you when they
look at you? In this experiment, we amplified what we did with our
mirror experiment. Each person in class paired up with a partner. We
instructed that, for this experiment, it was imperative for everyone to
resist the impulse to talk and that we needed to maintain silence. We
asked the students to sit in pairs, to get about seven to ten inches from
each other's face and to begin simply gazing at the other person or,
with a greater philosophical intent, to begin gazing at "the Other." We
held ourselves in that position for about five long minutes (in what felt
like an immensely charged and tense silence). We then asked that they
shift their state of mind a bit and attempt to look at the Other *as an
object*. We suggested that they focus on the eyeball of the Other as an
object, as a physical entity as opposed to a form of personal contact,
to notice the eyeball's color, texture, veins, movements, and the like—
almost like an ophthalmologist's gaze. We suggested that they focus on
the *biology* of the Other. After two minutes of this, we then specifically
instructed them to mentally adjust and to feel themselves *looked at* as
an object by the Other-as-subject. Then again, after an eternally long,
short while (two minutes), we asked them to mentally flip this over
and once again to simply resume gazing at the Other. After holding
this entire situation for 10 minutes, we all closed our eyes for about a
minute. Then we opened our eyes and, after another minute, we gently,
slowly, disengaged ourselves and immediately—still in silence--- wrote
out what we experienced. Finally, we lifted the "no talk" rule, and all
shared with their partner exactly what they experienced.

The Role of Thought

In this exercise, we are exploring the tension, the ordinary tension, *in* interaction, self/other interaction. On another level, we are also exploring the tension *of* interaction altogether (of not being alone on the planet, a singularity, but rather inhabiting-a-world-with-others).

What is the role of the *thought* of our appearance to the other in everyday interaction? This exercise strongly highlights this dimension of ordinary social interaction. As one student said, "All I kept thinking was 'What is this person thinking?'" Why do we think *knowing* what the other person is thinking gives us security and *not* knowing causes anxiety?

In this face-to-face silent encounter, all we can ever do is think *about* what the other is thinking: We can read and interpret their manifestation, appearance, and behavior, but we can't actually think their thoughts. Expanding on this situation, 99 percent of the time we're not perceiving the other's thoughts, we're projecting our own thoughts, and 99 percent of the time we're confusing our projections with perception.

So, we busy ourselves, day in, day out, anxious about what others are thinking ... about us. Suppose we were liberated from that internalized burden? We could instead relate directly to the other. We could also pay attention to what we are thinking and feeling without reference as to whether or not the other is also thinking and feeling that. We could be in the simple, clear presence of the other without cloud cover, without thoughts of the other's thoughts, without thought of the other as judge.

> *Theresa:* I don't exactly know why I was so uncomfortable with it, but I just felt really nervous. It was as though the other person could look inside of me through my eyes. I felt violated because they were in my space. They had crossed over the invisible red line each of us have drawn around ourselves. I felt as though the person looking into my eyes knew what I was thinking, feeling and experiencing.

> *David:* At first, I believe that I was afraid that my partner could look at me for a minute and because of that see the real me. There is a possibility that subconsciously I do not want anyone to see the real me. Then I

started to try to see the real her. I did this in an attempt to prove to myself that if I could see the real her, then she could see the real me. All I saw was an eyeball. Facial expressions had gone dead by this point, and all I saw was a face much like all the other faces in the world. This convinced me that she could not see into me, and I started to finally feel comfortable with the situation.

The Role of Norms

"It was like I just broke the law," one student remarked. This face-to-face experiment violates a host of subterranean norms that support ordinariness and normalness in everyday face-to-face interaction. Therefore, it makes these norms, these highly skilled and surgically precise methods we have of looking at each other, visible. We immediately and viscerally discover the "law of not staring" that we have all been so urgently and persistently socialized with. To not stare is by no means an instinctual format in our circuitry.

We're trained, apparently, to *not* look closely, to not look for more than a brief moment. It would appear that the normative rules and taboos of eye contact and eye control are designed to never allow us to examine things or be with things too closely or too intimately. In a sense, these rules foster ignoring rather than seeing.

The Role of Judgments

In terms of de-socialization, it is very important in this exercise that we *notice* the judgments of the critical voice. Many students say something along the lines of "I was looking at the other person's face (or, at my own face) and I started making all sorts of critical judgments about imperfections. Then I caught myself and got angry at myself because I shouldn't do that. I shouldn't be so critical." It's important to *notice* the critical judgments we are busily engaging in and *only to notice them*. This requires discipline, the discipline to simply notice them, rather than, as in the foregoing, to engage in *another* critical judgment on ourselves because we catch ourselves making so many critical judgments. In that moment of condemning ourselves for making so many critical judgments, in that feeling of guilt, we cease noticing our thought processes, our socialization, and re-submerge ourselves once again into the familiar, painful, and secure stream of judgments.

The Eye Object

In this face-to-face experiment, focusing in on the eye of the other brings about a new dimension of awareness.

> *Heather:* I noticed that it was easier to look at my partner's eye as an object because it took away the personal aspect of staring into him and instead allowed me to stare at him as if he were a thing rather than a person.

Unless we are ophthalmologists or somehow practicing the medical gaze, we rarely see the other's eyes as objects. When we actually do accomplish this, we cease seeing them as the support of a judgment that would reflect on our self. We instantaneously step right out of the world of ordinary social interaction. On some level, perhaps, we step outside the world of humanism and inter-subjectivity.

> *Brenda:* Treating the eyeball as an object was very easy for me. I effectively separated the eyeball from the person and looked at the mirror image of myself in its reflection. I wasn't worried about what I was thinking about what he was thinking about me as a moment before when he was looking into my eyes. I relaxed. I wasn't being evaluated, I wasn't evaluating.

According to Sartre's analysis of human inter-subjectivity in *Being and Nothingness*, it seems as though there is no middle ground: Either you are the observer or the observed—a subject psychologically commanding over an object or an object collapsed into self-consciousness submitting to a subject. This experiment, on the contrary, seems to conclude more along the lines of Heidegger's analyses in *Being and Time*, of humans experiencing the fellowship and communal boding of "being-with." There is that moment of calm that is finally reached when we stare long enough into each other's eyes. Momentarily we shed the onion layers of socialization and transcend the otherwise ceaseless, ordinary war of all against all. It is a moment, quite simply, of the recognition and acknowledgment of being. Beyond the Hobbesian war of subject verses object, we eventually find ourselves as the experience rather than the observer: the egoless recognition of our bedrock, mutual beingness. This is an experience of mutual being-there that is underneath and beyond all the fluctuations of nervousness about acceptance, rejection, and indifference, an experience that is prior to the cycles of desire, repugnance, and ignoring that are the ceaseless waves of the ocean of ordinary societal life. There is a moment beyond the wall of self. A moment of direct contact, more intimate and vulnerable perhaps than physical contact: existential contact, being-there-together. We experience an openness out onto the field of being beyond ego.

Another way of easily seeing that we are so obsessively concerned with how we look to others is to personally meet someone who isn't. Have you ever met anyone who unequivocally manifested loud and clear, yet with great kindness, gentleness, and no trace of aggression, that they were not at all concerned with how they appeared to others, with how they were being judged by others? Some have witnessed this with the Dalai Lama; some with Mother Theresa. Author McGrane's teacher, the Tibetan meditation master Chogyam Trungpa, Rinpoche had that quality. It was a shocking, inarticulate revelation that you knew when you came into his presence. He was just there; he was not there in the mode of ordinary concern or ordinary anxiety about what others were thinking about him. He was not there in any mode of anxiety whatsoever. Seeing that, and participating for a moment in that clear space, one had the unique opportunity to realize for the first time how truly deep, hidden in the background and all pervasive our familiar, ordinary anxiousness is.

Full-Body Gaze

As a further extension on the foregoing face-to-face exercise, we have also tried guiding students through a full-body gaze exercise. We've done this only after great trust, security, and seriousness of inquiry has been achieved in the classroom space. This exercise was also a further elaboration on our private Naked/Nude experiment with the mirror.

Again in total silence, we arranged them into male-female partners in two rows. We asked all the women to stand up and stare straight ahead, almost like a police lineup. We asked the seated men to slowly, beginning at the top of the head, run their eyes down, inch by inch, over the entire length of their partner's body down to the feet. "Behold the human form," we instructed. We then asked the women to turn around so their backs were toward their partners. The males, still sitting, were then asked to repeat the slow, detailed, full body gaze down the back of their partners to their feet. "Behold the human form." We then switched places, and the women sat down and slowly ran their gaze over the standing males, front side and back.

Robin: The worst part was when we had to stand up in front of each other and check each other out. I stood up first. This was not as difficult as I thought it would be. But when William stood up, I thought I was going to die. When it was time for him to look at my chest, I had to unlock my eyes from his. For some reason I felt bad, or naughty, for watching him look at me. I couldn't look back until I knew he had passed over the crotch area, too. When I looked at him from top to bottom, I had a problem with the crotch, and then the butt, two parts of the male anatomy I have never had a problem glancing at before. When guys aren't looking, I often catch myself sneaking a peek of a little behind. But somehow his watching my peeking made the experience completely different, to the point where it was not enjoyable anymore. The whole thing is very bizarre. I can't explain it!

Heather: As each inch of my body was gazed upon slowly and calculatingly, I felt anger and embarrassment well up inside of me. This personal experiment was beginning to feel like I do when I walk by a bunch of construction workers or a group of guys on the street. When they say the things they sometimes do and yell and whistle, I get so angry because I know they are scrutinizing my body in the same way—inch by inch. They don't know who I am inside, they just see my body as an object.

However, when it was my partner's turn to stand up and my turn to look him up and down, I felt completely different. To me it was no big deal and all I saw was a body. No perfections or imperfections, just a body. I wondered if he felt awkward or embarrassed or violated as I had. I was neither comfortable or uncomfortable looking at him, it was just a matter of fact. And it seemed to be much quicker and much more painless than when I was the one standing up.

It's interesting that in our society, we are socialized to judge and be judged so much based on appearances—yet we are not allowed nor encouraged to really scrutinize someone. This experiment highlighted the profound confusion in our judgmental society between being observed and being judged. It seems we fear being judged in the process of being observed. This experiment also often provoked insights into feminism and the politics of gender relations: For the first time, many men felt to a small degree how many women in our society daily feel.

Dan: When I looked at her from top to bottom I felt as if I were invading her in some way. She was standing directly in front of me. It was much different than looking at the nude photos of women. Of course, she wasn't naked but she wasn't a picture either. When my eyes came across the two no-no places I sped up my glance as if I were doing something wrong. The thought of actually looking at her breasts or her lower anatomy, even fully clothed, made me feel guilty, though I must admit that I have spent certain amounts of time gloating at nude pictures of women. In this personal instance it was much different. I had an easier time looking at her when her back was toward me. She was obviously still aware of what I was doing, but it was more like looking at a picture since she could not see me.

When she looked me over I wondered if she was thinking the same things I had. It was very awkward. I didn't like it at all. I didn't feel as if I were being admired. I felt like I was being judged on my superficial qualities.

Josh: As I began to scan her female body, I noticed that I was thinking of her as an object again. I felt a sense of embarrassment and was somewhat uncomfortable when I reached her eyes. This was because as I made eye contact with her we visually confirmed that I was just about to look over her entire body. I didn't want to offend Tiffany in anyway, yet at the same time I knew that she would not be able to see my eyes as I looked over certain parts of her body. Therefore, I freely observed Tiffany's female body with interest. The uncomfortable feeling of possibly invading Tiffany's body was eased when she was asked to turn around and I then looked at her body from the rear. During this, we made no eye contact so I was able to look at her body, and any of its certain parts with ease. Then it was my turn.

I, for the first time in this experiment, realized that I was also an object. Tiffany was using my body as an object to observe. The same feelings were aroused when Tiffany began to scan over my body yet I was on the other end. In addition, when I turned around, I knew that she could be looking at any part of my body she wanted, and I couldn't see her.

No Mirror: Reflecting on the Absence of Reflections

Why is it so important as an everyday practice to see what we look like? All day long, this periodic seeing of our reflections, this everyday senseless glancing into a mirror, pit stops at the well of Narcissus, adding fuel to the fires of self-conscious perception ... Why? Why is it so hard for us *not* to look in the mirror? Not to orient to our reflection? What if we eliminated them altogether?

The instructions for this exercise were to go cold-turkey. No mirrors. No reflections for an entire 24-hour day. Observe the symptoms of mirror-withdrawal and note what they reveal to you about your society, your self, and your habitual ways of being.

> *Louisa:* I feel blind. I don't know what I look like today. Everyone knows what I look like, yet I don't know myself.

> *Amanda:* Our compulsion to constantly assure ourselves of our existence by looking in the mirror relates to our uncertainty of who we really are.

> *Danielle:* I never realized how much I go out of my way to catch a reflection or glimmer of myself. It's like I constantly need reassurance.

Without the mirror, we feel as though we have just lost our face. When we are out in the wilderness for a few days, we soon forget we have a face. We become who we are, we become our face without reference to imagining its appearance to others, without the mirror preoccupation and the endless cycle of advertisements and reflections. Sontag has expressed well this relation to the face though she depicts it in reference to gender relations: "Women do not simply have faces, as men do; they are identified with their faces….a woman's face is potentially separate from her body. She does not treat it naturalistically. A woman's face is the canvas upon which she paints a revised, corrected portrait of herself" (Sontag 1979:470).

How we look becomes more primary and predominant than *what we see*. We become a visible exhibitionist object, imprisoning ourselves in our imagined appearances and locked in the circle of self-consciousness. Without the presence of the mirror, the presence of self-consciousness inside our consciousness greatly diminishes…after the initial withdrawal symptoms subside. (Before that, of course, we are a wreck, obsessing over how we look.) There is the world, the familiar world, and there are others in the world, period. The only thing missing is that curious ghost that we often do spend so much of our time concerned with called "how do I look to others?" There is now *only* the world and others—and now both these are much more vivid and real now that we are not *using* them to bounce and reflect back to us our image. There is a dramatic change in the texture of reality and the texture of our experience of that reality. It's like going from experiencing the world through the droning sonar system of a submarine endlessly emitting signals and closely monitoring feedback to finally surfacing and seeing the world directly with all its Technicolor texture.

Sonia: I felt like I was on a diet, of the worst kind, deprived of my dependence on the mirror. I believe, as was pointed out in the movie Ways of Seeing, that men look at women, and women look at themselves being looked at by men. Taking away the mirror, made going to work a traumatic event. Every time I saw a guy that I had my eye on, I would turn my head or escape … . What if there was no such thing as a mirror, or reflection, and people had no idea of what they looked like? I wonder if there would be so much pressure on appearance, or if personality would become more important than attractiveness. During the day I also wondered how much cumulative time is spent in the world in one year by women in comparison to men looking into mirrors.

8

UN-TV

No TV and Meditation TV

It is still possible to turn off the television set. It is no longer possible to turn off the television environment

(Goldsen 1977: 2).

There are times in life when the question of knowing if one can think differently than one thinks, and perceive differently than one sees, is absolutely necessary if one is to go on looking and reflecting at all

(Foucault 1985:8).

Sharon: The thing I can't figure out is why it is so addicting? Why will I watch the TV for hours when there aren't any shows on that I like. There must be something in the programs that is satisfying me. Perhaps it is the commercials that I am attracted to. They offer me all kinds of dreams of hope, beauty, and everlasting youth. And I do want those things and more. All these things I think when the TV is off. But when it's on I am in a dream state awaiting the next fantasy. Not all programs supply sufficient fantasy material but commercials certainly do. So, I think I watch TV for the advertising and not the programming itself. That's a little backwards and very frightening but I'm glad I realized that (just now).

Why Is It So Hard to Imagine the Elimination of Television?

Why does TV seem like a necessity? An absolutely unconquerable reality? Why does it *not* seem like a convention? Why does it feel more like a natural reality? When Mander titles his book *Four Arguments for*

the Elimination of Television, we can only blink incredulously. It's not four arguments to *stop* watching television but to *eliminate* television. What nonsense! Eliminate TV? Impossible! It sounds something like *"Four Arguments for the Elimination of Sex."* It's not going to happen. To even announce it is to show oneself aligned with the foolishly mad, the lunatic fringe. Why can't we, following Foucault, *think* the possibility of the elimination of television? Can we think the possibility of the elimination of radio? of telephones or cell phones? of computers? of the Internet? of money? of private property? How about of nuclear weapons? of armaments? of guns? That we can't think this possibility of the elimination of television, that we can't mentally envision it in a serious way as a possibility really signifies something. It shows, perhaps, that television is tied to our established structure of "what is possible" and "what is impossible," of "what could possibly happen" and "what just simply could never happen." We are in the presence of possibility— hence we are in the presence of imagination. We are also in the presence of our conception of "human nature"—what is and is not possible for humanity. We are in the presence of the politics of possibility and the human visionary imagination. Why can't we seriously entertain the possibility of eliminating television?

The Cigarette Century and the Television Century

When you first try to smoke a cigarette, the spontaneous response of your body is to cough violently, to spit and tear. You must somehow *suppress and override* this natural, bodily response to learn and train yourself to smoke. Very soon thereafter, you become a "professional" smoker, which is to say, you are well on your way to being addicted: You are addicted to the drug nicotine and to the delivery system we call "cigarettes." You are a smoker. Smoking affects all aspects of your life, and it also affects your relationship to others. It affects others in your physical environment—most dramatically and most seriously with "second-hand smoke"—a leading cause of cancer. We contend that there is a similar pattern, though in a very different form, with television, both direct and "second-hand television." As a child, your bodymind's first response to television is a subtle form of rejection. You visually wince somewhat, rather than cough, and you get both mesmerized and bewildered simultaneously. Soon thereafter, you become "professional," and often you become addicted.

Cigarette smokers pay for their addiction in the currency of their relationship to health. Health, for the smoker, becomes diminished. Their sense of smell atrophies, as does their sense of taste. In fact, all the dimensions of life shrink and atrophy, and the smoker adapts and adapts and adapts until he or she adapts him- or herself to sickness and death, somewhat like the infamous laboratory "frog experiment." In this laboratory experiment, a scientist drops a frog into a beaker of boiling hot water, and the frog immediately leaps out. A similar frog is then put into a beaker of comfortable, room-temperature water. At imperceptible degrees, the water is heated very slowly, one degree at a time. It goes up a degree, and the frog adapts. Ever so slowly it goes up another degree, and again the frog adapts. Another degree…and so on. Soon the frog has adapted itself to being boiled alive. We believe a somewhat similar phenomenon is happening to us in reference to our commercial TV media culture. Slowly we are marinating in and adapting to a dangerous cultural environment, we are *Amusing Ourselves to Death* (Postman 1985). Slowly our relationship to life is becoming anemic and atrophying.

For a moment, let us imaginatively put ourselves back into the situation of a cigarette smoker in the 1950s commercial media culture of denial. Let's say you have been smoking for 10 or 20 years. You started when you were about 12 or 13. You have some suspicions that all is not right, yet all the signs and messages from your culture, your media culture, assure you that cigarette smoking is essentially harmless. It is a minor indulgence, a small pleasure in life, something to reward yourself with. It is frequently glamorized. Everyone does it; it's cool. Alan Brandt's rigorous historic work, *The Cigarette Century: The Rise, Fall and Deadly Persistence of the Product that Defined America* (2007), analyzes this phenomenon thoroughly. This was the official commercial, corporate, media/advertising position for many, many decades—at least from the 1900s through the 1950s, 60s, and into the 70s (Bagdikian 1983, 2004).

Consider now the analogy with TV. It is essentially harmless. It is harmless to your health and well-being. At its worst, it is an indulgence; at its best, it is a positive advancement of the human enterprise: It is up there in the twentieth-century pantheon with the automobile, the telephone, the airplane, and the computer and Internet. Let's get paranoid just for a moment and suppose that there is a sort of anonymous cultural, media conspiracy to keep from you the fact that TV is bad for your health. TV stunts your growth and is addictive to your body-mind. It promotes mental enslavement to itself and its way of looking at the world.

The phenomenon of denial and resistance is paramount in most conversations regarding television. To be concerned about the health consequences of television is extremely difficult to "broadcast" to the society at large. Insofar as we are a member of this society, we are constrained to experience and think of TV as essentially benign, as essentially neutral, if not positive. In fact, in our current reality, we can no more object to the structural presence of TV in our media culture than we can object to the structural presence of English grammar in the English language that we speak. *This is just how it is.* To somehow question this is experienced as nonsensical and absurd.

In our reflections on television with our students, we have found it particularly perspicuous to engage ourselves with Mander's 1978 work, *Four Arguments for the Elimination of Television.* Reading Mander promotes some really seismic reflections on the cultural role and peculiar presence, the historical singularity, of television in our ordinary, familiar lives—for, on some level, the danger in television is not that it is there; it is that *we no longer notice it.* One of our students expressed some particularly honest feelings in this regard.

> *Rachel:* As I was reading these books I found myself much more attracted to *The Plug-In Drug* than to *Four Arguments for the Elimination of Television.* Yet I don't know whether my feelings about Mander's book have more to do with the way the book is written or with my innate discomfort with the topic of eliminating television. Mander says that the common reaction he got when people heard that he was writing a book advocating the elimination of television was an initial agreement followed by the question, "but you don't really expect to succeed do you?" (Mander 1978:347). He writes, "The people who asked [this question] had just admitted to hating television and yet I was left with the impression that they also hated the idea that I might actually believe it possible to get

rid of television" (Mander 1978:348). After reading that line, I realized that that issue, the sort of paradoxical attitude towards television, was the issue that made me uncomfortable with Mander. From the moment I read the title it made me uneasy. I am intelligent enough to recognize all the poisonous influence television has, yet at the same time I cannot imagine a world without it. This is probably largely due to the fact that I was one of those children who grew up with television as a third parent. I would probably feel uneasy reading a book called Four Arguments for the Elimination of Fathers as well. Yet appropriately enough, that belief, that eliminating television is impossible, is a very good illustration of Mander's argument for the elimination of television.

Mander in his work challenges us to imagine the elimination of television. Why does that challenge stop us? Why does it bring us up short? On the other side of this question, we also want to ask, "Why is it necessary to think about the possibility of the elimination of television? Why is it necessary to think of TV as *not* necessary?" Because this enterprise so relevantly and effectively goes against the grain of contemporary society, contemporary established reality. This topic, this approach yanks us—by its apparent absurdity—into the presence of our ideology, into the presence of our societal unconsciousness. The elimination of television is impossible. Period. It is the weight, the solidity of the "period" that needs to be explored. It sounds a bit like, "Ending war is impossible," period, or "Changing human nature is impossible," period. Is it possible to get to the other side of that period, to think to the other side of that period—to "think differently" as Foucault counsels. *What is the good of asking this question about the elimination of television?* What's the good of seeing it this way? *What's the good of choosing to see the elimination of television as impossible, rather than seeing it as possible?*

Can we imagine the elimination of television? In terms of addressing our epistemological awareness, we can, to use the Kantian technique, begin the imaginary process of elimination: We can imagine a world without people; we can imagine a world without animals, without plants, without life, and so on. We can imagine away item after item in the universe in this great cosmic, epistemological exercise in subtraction. Let us engage in subtraction to see whether there might be something that we cannot subtract away so that we may better be able to discover that which we cannot eliminate, that which transcends the process of elimination, of subtraction. We can imagine no earth; we can imagine no sun, no planets, no stars. We can imagine no matter in the universe. We are stopped when it comes to eliminating space and time. We can't imagine no space in the universe. We can't imagine a time when there is no time. In Kant's epistemological inquiry into the metaphysical foundations of reality, he effectively eliminated metaphysics. The Kantian turn of the Copernican revolution was that we can't imagine the nonexistence of space because space is not objective; it is not a distinct "entity." Space is in the structure of the imagining mind itself—though this is not to say that it is subjective. Space is the way through which we experience reality. It is a structural form, an apperception, of all experience and of all imagination. Because we can't eliminate space from our imaginings, it reveals itself as part of the very structure of imagining itself, and the same holds for time. Space is not an experienced object. Space is not objective—it is rather the very condition of reality, the condition of experience-ability and the condition of imaginativity. We cannot think without something to think with. We cannot think without space and time in the background as conditions making possible the very reality we are thinking within and about which we are thinking. Space and time are not items in reality—they are the very preconditions of reality. Space is neither objective nor subjective but rather that which makes possible the objective and the subjective. It is "a priori"—that which lies beneath and "before" all experience that makes experience possible. It "co-arises" with all experience.

In terms of our concern with critical reflections on the media, we would like to ask, for us, today, does television co-arise with all experience? For our modern historical situation, television does indeed seem to co-arise with all social experience. It has become a cultural a priori: That which is televised is real, that which is not televised is not real. That which is not televisable is not real and, of course, television cannot present the elimination of television.

There is a famous teaching in cultural anthropology called the *Sapir-Whorf* hypothesis. A central assertion of this hypothesis is that the language a person is socialized into dictates in profound and unconscious ways the very structure of reality. How we, then, experience the world is shaped less by how the world is and more by the filters that shape our experience: the grammar, syntax, semantic structure, lexicon, vocabulary, and texture of the language we have acquired. From this perspective, we live in different worlds depending on the deep structure of our acquired language. A key component of this anthropological teaching is that we as members of our culture don't notice that our experience of reality is *not* a direct experience of reality. This pre-structuring of our experience, this a priori filter, is unconscious to us. Even when we reflect upon it in a more conscious and direct way, we are *still employing it* in the analysis of it and hence are still in a sense confined and imprisoned by it.

We want to contend that our relationship to television has components deeply similar to those of the *Sapir-Whorf* hypothesis. Being socialized by television affects us as deeply, as indelibly, and as unconsciously as being socialized by language. From this perspective, learning how to watch television is learning a language, learning a skill that is similar to learning a language. Once we have acquired and internalized this language, we use it as a filter to look through and also as a means of communication, as a vehicle to speak through, to communicate with.

The language of television highlights certain aspects of reality and muffles other aspects. Famously it highlights dramatic moments and deeply muffles ordinary moments; it highlights excitement and entertainment and erases quiet stillness, boredom, and the mundane. Television helps us to *frame* our experience. It gives us a soundtrack, a surround soundtrack that continuously broadcasts, constantly seeping and dripping through the pores, the cracks and corners of reality as we know and experience it. Television perfumes our environment; everywhere today we encounter, subliminally, a sort of ever-present media fragrance.

Again, what if we ask, "What is the meaning of 'words'?" (Actually a good reflexive, analytic philosopher would insist that the question "What is the meaning of words" is, in fact, a nonsense question. It is an expression of confusion rather than a genuine philosophical question. We should rather say, "What is the meaning of the word *words*?") The very raising of this question assumes as secure and at hand, as transparent, the grasp of "meaning" and of "words" and, indeed, of language as a whole. In asking about the meaning of "words," we are already, always using words. We can't ask about the accomplishment of language without *always already using* language. We can't ask about objects in the world without using space and time. Language is a precondition, the hidden and assumed precondition that necessarily preconditions all inquiry and thinking about the nature of language. I think with words. *I* is a word. *Think* is a word. *With* is a word. *Words* is a word. *Is* is a word. "." is also, sort of, a word. All these background structures are present in each and every manifestation of inquiry, in each and every questioning—of course, *this one* included.

What of television? Is our life today all-pervasively permeated and conditioned by television? How has television come to be the great language game of the contemporary world? How has televisibility become the threshold to reality? We can't ask about a "show" in the same way we can't ask about a "word." All of television is present in each part of television in the same way that all of language is present in each part of it, in each word of it (including these words). We can imagine the elimination of various words, but we cannot imagine the elimination of language. Language is what enables me to do the eliminating, to imagine the eliminating. Similarly, television enables me to imagine eliminating various "shows" at the same time that television prevents me from imaginatively eliminating television. We can't imagine a world without television. Television is our contemporary language. Television has become our a priori. It has lodged in our imagination to such an irreversible extent that we can no longer imagine it no longer existing.

It would seem, then, that we are condemned to imagine television as existing, to see it as necessary. When any cultural form has achieved the status of a necessity, of "nature," it has truly triumphed into existence. For a historical contingency to have achieved the status and the position of a natural necessity is truly colossal.

As Freud said, any truly great event can no longer *be measured*, because it has become part of the fabric of the yardstick that *does the measuring*. We can't measure the impact of the establishment of television, nor of the transformation that it has wrought on the planet and on the reality of human life, because it is what we would be measuring that impact with. We would need to televise its impact for us—as a global human population—to truly *get* its impact. How do you measure a yardstick? How do you measure the impact of the emergence into being of language? What were we like before the invention of language? What were we like before the invention of television? What changes has the establishment of television brought about on the nature of human life? On the daily texture of human life and on the emotional relationship to reality that we have? How has television, the establishment of television, altered or affected our relationship to knowledge? How has television affected our relationship to the previous medium of knowledge, to books, to reading? To language itself?

"Reading a book" now is a completely different event-experience than it was before "watching television" emerged into human reality. The "*medium is the message*" has multiple dimensions and meanings to it. Reading in the age of television is totally different from reading in the Guttenberg galaxy, from reading in the age of the book. Likewise the computer-Internet dawning age is altering our experience of "watching television" and of "reading a book."

TV as the Most Powerful Force on the Planet

Suppose rather than eliminating television, we eliminate watching television. (As we have shown in many of our exercises, you can eliminate watching television by observing television.) This issue speaks to the heart of what we envision as socially possible. Yes, *we* can eliminate television in *our individual* personal life, but *we* can't eliminate television from *our* society. It's not going to happen. No way. The zone of interconnectedness between I and We is present here: what's possible for an "I" and yet what's not possible for a "We." What is at stake here is the foundation of *our* view of possibility.

"You can never end war, that's impossible." "You can't eliminate money, that's impossible." We are in the presence of the relation between the conventional and the natural, the artificial and the natural. Social agreements, social relations *can* be changed, can alter. Nature cannot. The entire Marxist, socialist movement of the last century and a half was grounded on the possibility of possibility. Behind social relations lies not nature but conventions. The conventions are grounded in ignorance, power, and exploitation. The root sociological ignorance is to *see the conventional as the natural.* To see the artificial as the inevitable. To see the created as the uncreated. When we do this, we are in the presence of "ideology," of pretending that things are the way they are by nature because it is inevitable rather than by human invention. *"You can't imagine a world without me" is the supreme accomplishment of television media ideology.* Pretending things are necessary that in fact are voluntary is the heart of ideology, of ignorance or the great pretence.

If you are able to get yourself to the position of envisioning the elimination of television, that in itself causes a transformation. Envision eliminating television in your life. Now envision eliminating television in the life of our society. To imagine this is to affect something, something in the deep structure of the landscape of possibility. To dwell in the possibility of that which has never been, and has never been imagined, is liberating.

Meditation Practice and Television Practice

We began this book by noting in Chapter One that the Dalai Lama practices meditation four hours a day. From the perspective of the Eastern paths of liberation, the nature of ego is "very professional" and overwhelmingly efficient in its own way. The renowned Tibetan meditation master Chogyam Trungpa has provided us with many vivid portraits of "ego."

> We need a very active and efficient mechanism to keep the instinctive and intellectual processes of ego coordinated. That is the last development of ego... Consciousness consists of emotions and irregular thought patterns, all of which taken together form the different fantasy worlds with which we occupy ourselves...the generals of ego's army; subconscious thought, day dreams and other thoughts connect one highlight to another. So thoughts form ego's army and are constantly in motion, constantly busy. Our thoughts are neurotic in the sense that they are irregular, changing direction all the time and overlapping one another. We continually jump from one thought to the next, from spiritual thoughts to sexual fantasies to money matters to domestic thoughts and so on. The whole development...is an attempt...to shield ourselves from the truth of our insubstantiality
>
> (Trungpa 1976:22–23).

TV programming is, like ego, very professional and overwhelmingly efficient in its own way. There are never any gaps on TV, never any periods when *nothing is happening*. What fundamentally is this all about? In terms of the conventional, ordinary television trance, this fear of nothing happening is the fear of the spell being broken. The seamless flow, highly professional and immensely managed down to the microsecond, would be interrupted. The perpetual-motion machine would halt. From the programmers' perspective, this interruption is seen and experienced as panic, as breakdown, as the great threat to be avoided at all costs. It would not even remotely be considered as a cordial moment of simple human silence, a brief opening and gesture toward the background of being related and being together.

Consider that there are, let us say, two experiences of silence. When two or more people are having the experience of being close, comfortable, relaxed, and familiar with each other, they can let silence be: They can let silence be in the midst of their interaction, their conversation. This is a becalming silence. When people are having a suppressed, estranged, and anxious experience with each other, there is, in contrast, a loud, threatening, and ominous view of silence: "My God! We're going to be revealed, negatively, to each other. Quickly! Quickly! Rush in and say something! Fill up the silence." TV, obviously, lives in our culture entirely in the silence-as-threat camp. It reinforces this perspective deep in its structure. Silence doesn't make good TV.

We could say that behind television entertainment lies anxiety. Anxiousness about not-being-entertained lies just below the surface of this televisual entertainment culture. and this anxiousness continuously threatens to break out at any moment, like a shark fin suddenly breaking the calm surface. In this sense, television entertainment conceals anxiety. This *form of entertainment* conceals anxiety rather than offering itself as an artistic expression, an exuberance and overflowingness. If this form of entertainment conceals anxiousness, it also perpetuates and reinforces the very anxiousness that its function is to conceal. From this angle, commercial TV programming needs anxiousness to function and, hence, we might say serves to keep anxiousness alive and well in our overall culture.

There is a tremendous amount of brilliant planning, design, and control to professionally manage and maintain this intensely efficient machinery. There is no passivity in the production of this entertainment passivity. It is grimly intense and highly focused. We'd wager it is at least as brilliantly and professionally planned, managed, and executed as any of the large-scale space flights that NASA puts on.

In the Eastern paths of meditation practice, you vividly see the highly professional administration and bureaucracy of your ego. In the process of sitting quietly and just attentively being with your mind and labeling your thoughts "thinking" with as much precision, accuracy, and gentleness as you can, you become keenly aware that your mind compulsively thinks all the time. There is that little voice, that internal conversation and stream of subconscious gossip that just goes on and on virtually incessantly. It often drives beginning meditators crazy to realize how non-stop and totally out-of-control our "monkey-mind" actually is. In seeking silence, mental silence, in attempting to have an inner peace and stop talking to ourselves for a few moments, we unambiguously experience in the medium of our mind how nonexistent real "dead air time" is. The "voice" or the "committee" goes on incessantly despite all efforts to simply "turn it off." In a manner of speaking, the television is permanently "on" in our inner proscenium. The "on/off" button or even the "mute" button seems nowhere to be found...ever.

When we meditate, we can easily and relatively quickly encounter panic in this initial confrontation with the compulsive broadcasting chatter of our jumpy, discursive minds. We thought we could stop thinking at will. We thought we had control over our own thinking. We thought we could *not think* that we could *stop thinking*. We soon realize we don't have control and we can't stop. We're ready to join "thinkers anonymous." During this phase of panic on the path of meditation, we access the anxiousness below the surface of our compulsive thinking. All along, there has been this anxiousness regarding "dead air time"— nothing happening, no entertainment, time passing. The bureaucracy and administration of ego is structurally driven in a deeply analogous way to the bureaucracy and administration of commercial television-radio and now also Internet programming. Behind and beyond the commercial practicality of the enterprise, covering and calming anxiousness and "dis-ease" is the task and the function. "...you are always already ready for the next show, even before this one is over" (deZingotita 2006:17). We compulsively talk to ourselves to avoid being and to avoid silence; and we compulsively watch TV to entertain, sootheand distract our anxiousness.

Television Versus Meditation

Let us contrast the experience of television with the experience of meditation. With meditation, we see thoughts arise and dwell and disappear. We hear ourselves talking to ourselves. Or, we might say, we hear our voice talking: We hear murmuring conversations. We notice these conversations. They arise, dwell momentarily, and vanish. Sometime later, we can often recognize that we are also the silence, the all-encompassing volume of silence, of space, within and through which these conversations happen. There is a great variety to these conversations: monologues, staged dialogues between self and other (almost all invented), memories, future plans, intense multiparty conversations generated by what seems "a committee" inside our heads. In meditation practice, we alternate back and forth between identifying with these conversations and becoming mindful and noticing these conversations, between being lost in these conversational dreams and dramas and not being lost in them, between being asleep inside these conversations and waking up to them, between being unconscious and being conscious. We actually experience silence, the absence of anything being said, and the absence of commentary. We become absolutely present, here, now. One some basic level, we experience ordinary "enlightenment."

With television, we are absorbed inside the entertainment. The voice, the dialogue, the drama captivate us. The ordinary stream of subconscious gossip that we personally have appears momentarily to be silenced, but actually it is shoved so far to the back of our inner proscenium that we no longer notice it. We are noticing the show, not our chattering mind. That doesn't mean that our chattering mind is stopped or liberated into the environmental, sane energy of awareness but rather that it is heavily suppressed and driven underground—very similar to what happens on certain drugs.

TV, as Mander maintains in *Four Arguments for the Elimination of Television*, is sleep teaching. What is the somatic situation of television? Our body is still. We can't really be physically active and fully absorb television media simultaneously. The circumambient universe must be dimmed out, darkened. It just doesn't work to watch TV out of doors, say, in the middle of a meadow on a beautiful day. TV is always an "affair of the night." It's always in darkened rooms—even when the room is full of natural or artificial light, it is still a darkened environment, a cave. On one level, we love TV because it makes all our cares go away. It allows us to vegetate, to "relax" or "veg" as we say. One of us, McGrane, remembers to this day how he noticed many years ago that as his grandfather was dying of cancer at home, his family built a stand to set the TV up high on the wall, like in the hospital rooms, so he could experience some comfort and escape from his pain. The comfort and escape we create with TV is as it is—not good, not bad. The quality, degree, and amount of comfort and escape are the issue. The statistics remain steady: four hours a day, seven days a week. To be engaged in watching TV is to not be engaged in other activities.

We escape from our own lives. We escape from life. When we are inside media land, we are not present to life. When we are inside meditation, we are present to our life. We are present to our life individually speaking and also universally speaking. We are present to our own individual life, and we are also present to life per se—to the life that goes on within us and without us. We are present to the life within us, to "my life," yet simultaneously we are present to the life without us, that is to say, to life without the "me" in it, to life as life—and hence also to life with a capital L: to Life. This includes my life and my death—the present existence of me and the eventual death of me, the end of my life, the life going on in the particular form that is me, that is "I" and that is "you."

> Our usual understanding of life is dualistic: you and I, this and that, good and bad. But actually these discriminations are themselves the awareness of the universal existence. "You" means to be aware of the universe in the form of you, and "I" means to be aware of it in the form of I
>
> (Suzuki 1970:29).

In meditation practice, we can achieve what the Buddhist's call "right view." We see our proper proportion. It is a profoundly humbling experience, similar to what we get when we go into the wilderness, out onto the ocean, or simply look up at the stars and try to announce our own self-importance to the cosmos. We immediately get accurate feedback as to our own importance in the scheme of things.

Our current national practice of "television meditation"—four hours a day, seven days a week—doesn't give us access to any of that. In fact, it reverses most of it. In television world, human life is of primary importance and concern. Only human life is of interest. Commercial television is anthropomorphic down to the last molecule. Also, there is no death on television. While we engage in the practice of television meditation, we can't really access or relate with death, impermanence, or mortality. Yes, indeed, there is the spectacle of death, but that is death experienced inside the insulating form of entertainment, death experienced against the background of fascination, curiosity, and exhilaration, death-as-entertainment: "Ha! Whew! It was them-and-not-me. It was their death—something that *could* happen to them. It is without direct reference to me and my life."

TV, Meditation Practice, and the River of Thoughts

The issue we want here to look at is the actual process by which we lose ourselves into the TV, the hypnotic quality of the medium and the way it parallels meditation practice. In meditation practice, we become aware that we are lost in the samsaric projections of our thought processes. As we mentioned earlier, we talk to ourselves continuously, our stream of consciousness/subconsciousness, our stream of conversations are ongoing and seemingly without break, a seamless flow. As there is never a break in the flow of a river, where suddenly the water stops, where there is a "gap," a space of non-water in the river water, so likewise it seems as if there is never a gap in the flowing current of our thoughts-and-feelings. Because of this ancient uninterruptedness of flow, we deeply identify with it and take it to be real: That is to say, we do not recognize it as a flow of thoughts, as discursive thoughts and feelings ongoingly streaming into being, ongoingly arising, dwelling, and evaporating. Somewhere, there occurs a gap during the actual process of meditation practice when abruptly there are no thoughts. For a brief moment, the humming, droning machine of conversations stops, and there is an opening out onto silence, onto space, onto being. Then again, the river of language flows back in upon itself and there is commentary: "Oh, I just experienced a moment of silence; I just experienced a moment without commentary." We're watching this river flow by, and suddenly there is this abrupt, distinct negative space of no water. We recognize it by the boundaries of water all around in contrast with which it clearly is non-water, non-thought. Then in an instant, willy-nilly, the water rushes in from all sides to fill up this vacuum, this momentary experience of "sunyata" or emptiness (emptiness here means empty of concepts). After enough of these experiences, these meditative realizations, we become aware of the river water itself in a way that we could not have done before. Instead of "all that is," it becomes a unique, identifiable "substance." We recognize the river water *as* river water. It becomes river water in contrast to the non-river-water. Whereas before it just *was*, now it is identifiable as a specific entity, as river water.

This process is similar to what happens in both the gradual and the sudden discovery that our thoughts are just... thoughts. We think we are face to face with reality and, it turns out, we are face to face with our thoughts, with our-thoughts-appearing-as-reality. Through these shifts and shocks, we slowly awaken to recognizing our thoughts as *not being reality*. This actually is a big step for someone practicing meditation; the very ground and relationship to reality shifts and moves. (It's sort of like the moment of recognizing this 10-dollar bill as being a piece of paper. It is not money in itself, it is not value in itself.)

What we are watching on TV is not reality. We thought we were face to face with reality, and yet it turns out that we were not. We thought reality was a story, a drama, and was actually accompanied by a musical score. We now see the TV and the show in a way that we never have before. It becomes broken down into the photographs it is composed of. We can now recognize the technical events. We can see the brilliant or mediocre artistry with which it was composed. We can see that it *is* composed. It is an artificial construction of reality designed above all to *not* be recognized as an artificial construction of reality. Its artificialness must be folded and tucked into itself so as not to draw attention to itself. The best edits are those we are unconscious of. If, in watching the photo, we say to ourselves "That is beautiful," it is successful. If we say, "That is a beautiful photo," it fails. We are unconscious of whatever medium we are exposed to at the moment.

Cinema, Time, and the Eternal Present: Going Back into the Cave?

If we are to some degree liberated from the cave and to some degree free of the confines of the cave, if we are out wandering in the fields of reality, *should we go back to the cave?* Should we go back to visit? To tell others about our experience so that they too may leave if they so choose? Or, rather should we wall up the cave?

No. Rather than all that, we should go to a movie. Plato, and many, many after him, was deeply suspicious of the impact of art, of the influence of art on the rational mind. He would, I'm sure, be very dubious of the irresistible swept-away quality of our contemporary cinema. The film gives us access to a realm of intensity, an exposure to emotional vulnerability that is perhaps without precedence in the history of art. We want to contend that *when we watch a film, we are on some level voluntarily going back down into the cave.*

> If you really appreciate an object of beauty, then you completely identify with it and forget yourself. It is like seeing a very interesting, fascinating movie and *forgetting that you are the audience.* At that moment there is no world; your whole being is that scene of that movie
>
> (Trungpa 1973:16; emphasis ours).

The nature of the media immersion is most fascinating. How is it that we suspend disbelief in a radical and profound way and forget that we are the audience? We suspend disbelief by engaging in a sort of hyper-identification. What happens when we go into the movie theatre? We take our seat. We sit. It would be a very different experience if we stood. Body posture and bodily choreography are so important and so invisible—so non-present and disattended to. We settle into rest mode, to meditative stillness. Again, it would be a very different experience if we were to walk about—sort of like the experience of the art museum. We sit in stillness. We cease talking to others. We cease listening to others. Soon into the movie, we cease listening to our self. (In meditation, we sit still in silence and listen to the unceasing stream of conversations "in our mind.") We look forward at the screen. The images begin, the moving pictures and sound and willy-nilly we are swept away into another world, living someone else's life. We are "riding the movies." Within a few moments we are completely immersed in the present-moment-spectacle. We are completely oblivious to what is outside the movie theatre. What is going on in the lobby? We are no longer present to what was troubling us during the day nor to what concerns we have about tomorrow. *We are transported into the present, into the spectacle.* We identify with what we are seeing and hearing. We *are* the spectacle we are seeing and hearing. Perhaps the only other depth psychology dimension of mental life analogous to this total, cinematic, media immersion is the phenomenon of dreaming. We produce, or perhaps "manifest," the dream world—the spectacle, the characters, the action, the narrative story, the soundtrack. We are in it, and yet we also get to observe it as a spectator simultaneously. In the dream, we are the projector, and we are the theatre and the screen, and we are the film being projected, the character on the screen and the audience watching. There is a sheer, all-encompassing, overwhelming presence, a complete identification and a total forgetting of our ordinary, everyday, wide-awake conscious reality.

Time is suspended. Actually our "I" is suspended. We experience a time outside of time. We are relieved of the burden of being our self—the burden of being a troubled, slightly anxious, fidgety, discontented human being. A component of this experience is that we are endeavoring to push our self through the membrane of time into the eternity of the present. Our normal psychological machinery of anticipating the future, of being-towards-the-future, of being guided by the future-we-are-living-into is completely suspended. While we are immersed in the film, we don't feel that this feeling of total identification will be over in two hours, as then we would be subconsciously or "laterally" aware of anticipating the future and of "time-passing." The whole enormous seduction of the film is that it deeply and radically annihilates time.

We step into the cinema, and our sense of the weight and viscosity of time passing is instantly altered. We step into an altered reality in that sense. When we alter the lived experience of the flow of time, we alter reality. Take any significant psychoactive drug, and one of the foundational psychic transformations that happens is in the realm of the lived experience of time. When time is suspended, when we enter a time away from time, we enter an altered reality. When we are in the mode and mood of struggling distractedness, we are distractedly aware of the slow passage of time. We blink and look away. When we are completely absorbed and at one with what we are doing, we are also at one with time-flow. To be at one with time is in a sense to be in eternity—the eternity of the present moment, or the eternity of nowness. Cinema is instant nowness, instant pre-packaged eternity.

When we watch a film, we are not mentally struggling. There is no attention deficit disorder occurring—we are *all attention*. We are continuous present-moment attention. There is no future. There is no past. There is no "me." There is only the sheer event that is going on. Perhaps in some obscure yet real sense, in the realm of art, to watch film is to experience enlightenment. The quality of the eternal present is at the heart of the magic of the art of cinema, and in that sense the cinema is about eternity: "If we take eternity to mean not infinite temporal duration but timelessness, then eternal life belongs to those who life in the present" (Wittgenstein 1961:147). The cinema is the cathedral of access into the present moment. It functions as the artistic salvation of our ordinary troubled consciousness. Those on the screen, the celebrities, not those responsible for creating the film (the directors) are the gods of salvation. (Their faces are 20 to 40 feet tall: They must be gods. Think of the infants gazing up at the enormous, colossal figure of its parent, the infantile experience of the actual awe of god. In the cinema, we are in an infant's size range in reference to the large persons we are gazing at on the Giant Screen and, hence, we are in infant-toned awe at these colossal figures.)

When we are watching a film, we can notice that we are absorbed out onto the film to such a degree that we momentarily cease to be aware of our stream of subconscious gossip, our stream of conversational consciousness. We cease to be aware of our anxiousness, our all pervasive ordinary anxiousness, and we become absorbed in the spectacle, the drama, the technical wizardry of the rapid-fire, relentless, magical perspectives of the camera. If you find yourself saying "Look how beautiful that background scene is, like a great landscape painting," you are consciously noticing it, and you are not in the aesthetic presence of "great art." To be "in the presence of great art," you must be, in a sense, bludgeoned into unconsciousness as Nietzsche addressed in The Birth of Tragedy (1967). The good edit is the one you are unaware of. The good angle, the good background is the one you are unaware of. To be consciously watching the film is not to be within the art dimension of the film. That is to say, you are in contact not with the film as art but rather with the craft of the art. Art, like dreams, requires that we surrender our agency-consciousness to it. We must surrender our consciousness into the unconsciousness of art, the artistic experience.

We are reminded here of Lao Tsu and his comments on government and on ruling. The best ruler is one that no one notices. The second best is one that people love. The third best is one that people fear, and the worst is the ruler that people despise. The greatest films are not noticed as films—in the alchemical, aesthetic magic of experiencing them, they register indelibly as more than reality. In films we consciously surrender to the illusion and leave the reality of everyday life. Growing up and living in the world of the consumer media matrix of today that choice does not exist. Until we realize the hold television culture has on our reality we surrender to its whims without being aware.

> "Then we must apply this image, my dear Glaucon," said I, "to all we have been saying. The world of our sight is like the habitation in prison…the ascent and the view of the upper world is the rising of the soul into the world of mind … but God knows if it is really true… ."
>
> (*The Republic* 517B).

Bibliography

Alcoholics Anonymous: Big Book, 4th Edition. 2002. New York: Alcoholics Anonymous World Services, Inc.

Alexie, S. 2007. *Flight: A Novel.* New York: Grove Press, Black Cat.

Andrejevic, M. 2004. *Reality TV: The Work of Being Watched.* Lanham, MD: Rowman & Littlefield.

Bagdikian, B. 1983. *The Media Monopoly.* Boston: Beacon Press.

Bagdikian, B. 1990. *The Media Monopoly*, 3rd edition. Boston: Beacon Press.

Bagdikian, B. 2004. *The New Media Monopoly.* Boston: Beacon Press.

Berger, J. 1972. *Ways of Seeing.* New York: Penguin Books.

Berger, P., and Luckman, T. 1966. *The Social Construction of Reality.* New York: Anchor Doubleday.

Bierce, A. 1911. *The Devil's Dictionary.* New York: Dover Publications.

Bourdieu, P. 1998. *On Television.* New York: The New Press.

Brandt, A. 2007. *The Cigarette Century: The Rise, Fall, and Deadly Persistence of a Product that Defined America.* New York: Basic Books

Buber, M. 1970. *I and Thou.* New York. Charles Scribner's Sons.

Carnes, P. 2001. *Out of the Shadows: Understanding Sexual Addiction.* Center City, MN: Hazelden.

Castaneda, C. 1972. *Journey to Ixtlan.* New York: Pocket Books.

Collingwood, R. G. 1956 *The Idea Of History.* London: Oxford University Press.

Daly, M. 1978. *GYN/Ecology: The Metaethics of Radical Feminism.* Boston: Beacon Press.

DeBord, 1967. *The Society of the Spectacle.* Detroit. Black and Red.

de Zengotita, T. 2005. *Mediated: How the Media Shapes Our World and the Way We Live in It.* Bloomsbury USA.

Eco, U. [1973]1990. *Travels in Hyperreality.* New York: Harcourt.

Elgin, D. 1990. "Television and the Environment." *Adbusters Quarterly.* Vol. 1, No. 3. pp. 10–11.

Ehrenreich, B. 1990. *The Worst Years of Our Lives: Irreverent Notes from a Decade of Greed.* New York: Pantheon Books.

Ewen, S. 1988. *All Consuming Images.* New York: Basic Books.

Fogel, R. W., and Engerman, S. L. 1974. *Time on the Cross: The Economics of American Negro Slavery.* Boston: Little, Brown and Company.

Foucault, M. 1985. *The History of Sexuality, Vol. 2: The Use of Pleasure.* New York: Vintage.

Fox, Emmet, 1934. *The Sermon On The Mount.* New York: Harper and Brothers

Fromm, E. 2001. *The Fear of Freedom*. London: Routledge Classics.

Freud, Sigmund [1928] 1964 *The Future of an Illusion*. New York: W.W. Norton

Freud, S. 1955. *Moses and Monotheism*. New York: Vintage

Freud, S. 1962. *Totem and Taboo*. New York: W. W. Norton

Garfinkel, H. 1967. *Studies in Ethnomethodology*. Englewood Cliffs, NJ: Prentice Hall.

Gass, W. 1971. *Fiction and the Figures of Life*. Boston: Nonpareil.

Gitlin, T. 1986. *Watching Television*. New York: Pantheon.

Gitlin, T. 2002. *Media Unlimited: How the Torrent of Images and Sounds Overwhelms Our Lives*. New York: Holt Paperbacks.

Goffman, E. 1959. *Presentation of Self in Everyday Life*. New York: Anchor Doubleday.

Goldsen, 1977. *The Show and Tell Machine*. Dial Press

Gurdjieff, G. I. 1969. *Meetings with Remarkable Men*. New York: E. P. Dutton.

Hanh, Thich Nhat. 1992. *Peace is Every Step*. New York: Bantam

Heidegger, M. 1962. *Being and Time*. New York: Harper & Row.

Heritage, J. 1984. *Garfinkel and Ethnomethodology*. Cambridge, UK: Polity Press.

Inaba D.E. and Cohen W. E., 2005. *Upper, Downers, All Arounders: Physical and Mental Effects of Psychoactive Substances*. Medford, OR: CNS Publications.

Irwin, William 2002. *The Matrix And Philosophy: Welcome To The Desert Of The Real*. Chicago, IL: Open Court Press.

Jaynes, J. 1976. *The Origin of Consciousness and the Breakdown of the Bicameral Mind*. Boston: Houghton Mifflin Company.

Kierkegaard, S. 1980. *The Sickness Unto Death*. Princeton, NJ: Princeton University Press.

Kilbourne, J. 1977. Images of Women in TV Commercials. In J. Fireman (Ed.), *TV Book*. New York: Workman Publishing Co.

Kilbourne, J. 1999. *Can't Buy My Love: How Advertising Changes the Way We Think and Feel*. New York: Touchstone.

Klosterman, C. 2004. *Sex, Drugs, and Cocoa Puffs: A Low Culture Manifesto*. New York: Scribner.

Kosimar, L. 1971. The Image of Women in Advertising. In V. Gornick and B. Moran (Eds.), *Women in Sexist Society*. New York: Basic Books.

Kowinski, B. 1993. Graven Images. *Adbusters Quarterly*. Vol. 2, No. 3.

Life Magazine. 1992. *TV Guide Poll*. p. 26.

Lorenz, K. 1982. *The Foundations of Ethnology: The Principle Ideas and Discoveries in Animal Behavior*. New York: Touchstone.

Macionis, J. J. and Benokratis, N. V. 1989. *Seeing Ourselves*. Upper Saddle River, NJ: Prentice Hall.

Mander, J. 1978. *Four Arguments for the Elimination of Television*. New York: Quill.

Mander, J. 1991. *In the Absence of the Sacred*. San Francisco, CA: Sierra Club Books

McPherson, M., Smith-Lovin, and Brashears, M.E .2006. Social isolation in America: Changes in Core Discussion Networks over Two Decades. *American Sociological Review Vol. 71, No. 3*. June 2006. pp. 353–375.

McKenna, T. 1993. *Food of the Gods: The Search for the Original Tree of Knowledge A Radical History of Plants, Drugs, and Human Evolution.* New York: Bantam.

McKibben, B. 1992. *The Age of Missing Information.* New York: Random House

McLuhan, E., and Zingrone, F. 1995. *Essential McLuhan.* New York: Basic Books.

McLuhan, M. 1962. *The Gutenberg Galaxy: The Making of Typographic Man.* New York: New American Library.

McLuhan, M. 1964. *Understanding Media: The Extensions of Man.* New York: New American Library

McLuhan, M., Bernedetti, P., DeHart, N., Zingrone, F., and Marchand, P. 1996. *Forward Through the Rearview Mirror: Reflections on and by Marshall Mcluhan.* Cambridge, MA: The MIT Press.

Mead, G. H. 1962. *Mind, Self, and Society.* Chicago: University of Chicago Press.

Mendizza, M., and Pearce, J. C. 2003. *Magical Parent Magical Child, the Optimum Learning Relationship.* Nevada City, NV: In-Joy Publication.

Meyrowitz, . 1985. *No Sense of Place: The Impact of Electronic Media on Social Behavior.* New York: Oxford University Press USA.

Miller, J. 1971. *Marshall McLuhan.* New York: The Viking Press

Miller, P. W. 2000. *Nonverbal Communication in the Workplace.* Chicago, IL: Patrick W Miller & Associates.

Mills, C. W. 1956. *The Power Elite.* London: Oxford University Press.

Nietzsche, F. [1872] 1967. *The Birth of Tragedy.* Translated by Walter Kaufman York: Random House.

Nietzsche, F. [1887] 1967. *On the Genealogy of Morals.* Translated by Walter Kaufman. New York: Random House.

Palmer, P. 1998. *The Courage to Teach: Exploring the Inner Landscape of Teacher's Lives.* Jossey-Bass

Packard, V. [1957] 1980. *The Hidden Persuaders.* New York: Pocket.

Parenti, M. 1986. *Inventing Reality: The Politics of the Mass Media.* New York: St. Martin's Press

Parenti, M. 1992. *Make Believe Media: The Politics of Entertainment.* New York: St. Martin's Press.

Plato 2003. *The Republic.* New York: Penguin Classics

Postman, N. 1985. *Amusing Ourselves to Death: Public Discourse in the Age of Show Business.* New York: Penguin.

Putnam, R. D. 2000. *Bowling Alone: The Collapse of the American Community.* New York: Simon and Schuster.

Ray, V. 1984. *Advertising the Contradictions.* Berkeley, CA: Violet Ray.

Sartre, J. P. [1943]1969. *Being and Nothingness.* London: Routledge Classics.

Scheuer, J. 1999. *Sound Bite Society: Television & the American Mind.* New York: Four Walls Eight Windows.

Schudson, M. [1984]1986. *Advertising, the Uneasy Persuasion: Its Dubious Impact on American Society.* New York: Basic Books.

Slater, P. 1990. *The Pursuit of Loneliness.* Boston: Beacon Press.

Sontag, S. 1979. The Double Standard of Aging. In J. Williams (Eds.), *Psychology of Women: Selected Readings.* New York: W.W. Norton and Company.

Steinem, G. 1993. *Revolution from Within: A Book of Self-Esteem*. Boston, MA: Little, Brown and Company.

Sutton-Smith, B. 1971. "Children at Play," *Natural History*, Special Supplement, Play, December, Vol LXXX, No. 10, pp. 54–9.

Suzuki. 1970. *Zen Mind, Beginners Mind: Informal Talks on Zen, Meditation and Practice*. Boston, MA: Shambala.

Thomas, W., and Thomas, D. 1928. *The Child in America*. New York: Knopf.

Tolle, Eckhardt 2005. *A New Earth: Awakening To Your Life's Prupose*. New York: Plume.

Trungpa, C. 1973. *Cutting Through Spiritual Materialism*. Boston, MA : Shambhala.

Trungpa, C. 1976. *The Myth of Freedom. and the Way of Meditation*. Boston, MA: Shambhala.

Wallace, D. F. 1997. *A Supposedly Fun Thing I Will Never Do Again: Essays and Arguments*. San Francisco: Back Bay Books.

Wachtel, P. L. 1989. *The Poverty of Affluence: A Psychological Portrait of the American Way of Life*. Philadelphia, PA: New Society Publishers.

Williamson, J. 1978. *Decoding Advertisements: Ideology and Meaning in Advertising*. London and New York: Marion Boyars.

Winn, M. 2002. *The Plug-In Drug: Television, Computers, and Family Life*. 25th anniversary edition. New York: Penguin.

Wittgenstein, L. [1921] 1961. *Tractatus Logico-Philosophicus*. London: Routledge and Kegan Paul.

Wolf, N. 1991. *The Beauty Myth: How Images of Beauty are Used Against Women*. New York: William Morrow and Company.

Permissions

The authors and publisher are grateful for permission to use the following material in this book.

Preface

Excerpt from *The Matrix* written by Laurence "Larry" Wachowski and Andrew Paul "Andy" Wachowski. Courtesy of Warner Bros. Entertainment Inc. Copyright © 1999.

Chapter 1

Reprinted with permission from the *Diagnostic and Statistical Manual of Mental Disorders*, Text Revision, Fourth Edition, (© 2000 American Psychiatric Association).

Extracts from *Amusing Ourselves To Death* by Neil Postman, © 1985 Neil Postman. Used by permission of Viking Penguin, a division of Penguin Group (USA) Inc.

Chapter 2

© The New Yorker Collection 1974. Al Ross from cartoonbank.com. All rights reserved.

Excerpts from *Four Arguments for the Elimination of Television* by Jerry Mander. © 1978 Jerry Mander. Reprinted by permission of HarperCollins Publishers.

From *The Age of Missing Information* by Bill McKibben, © 1992 Bill McKibben. Used by permission of Random House, Inc.

Extracts from *The Plug-In Drug*, Revised and Updated 25th Anniversary Edition by Marie Winn, © 1977, 1985, 2002 Marie Winn Miller. Used by permission of Viking Penguin, a division of Penguin Group (USA) Inc.

Chapter 3

Excerpts from *Four Arguments for the Elimination of Television* by Jerry Mander. © 1978 Jerry Mander. Reprinted by permission of HarperCollins Publishers.

From *The Age of Missing Information* by Bill McKibben, © 1992 Bill McKibben. Used by permission of Random House, Inc.

Extracts from *Reality TV: The World of Being Watched* by Mark Andrejevic. Reprinted by permission of Rowman & Littlefield. Copyright © 2003.

Chapter 4

Excerpts from *Four Arguments for the Elimination of Television* by Jerry Mander. © 1978 Jerry Mander. Reprinted by permission of HarperCollins Publishers.

Extracts from *Reality TV: The World of Being Watched* by Mark Andrejevic. Reprinted by permission of Rowman & Littlefield. Copyright © 2003.

Extracts from *The Plug-In Drug*, Revised and Updated 25th Anniversary Edition by Marie Winn, © 1977, 1985, 2002 Marie Winn Miller. Used by permission of Viking Penguin, a division of Penguin Group (USA) Inc.

Chapter 5

Reprinted with the permission of Scribner, a division of Simon & Schuster, Inc., from *Sex, Drugs & Cocoa Puffs: A Low Culture Manifesto* by Chuck Klosterman. © 2003 Chuck Klosterman. All rights reserved. Also used by permission of James Levine Communications, Inc.

Extracts from *Amusing Ourselves To Death* by Neil Postman, © 1985 Neil Postman. Used by permission of Viking Penguin, a division of Penguin Group (USA) Inc.

Extracts from *The Plug-In Drug*, Revised and Updated 25th Anniversary Edition by Marie Winn, © 1977, 1985, 2002 Marie Winn Miller. Used by permission of Viking Penguin, a division of Penguin Group (USA) Inc.

Chapter 6

Extract from *Playboy* March 1963 "Playboy Interview: Marshall McLuhan". Reprinted by permission of Playboy Enterprises, Inc.

Extracts from *The Plug-In Drug*, Revised and Updated 25th Anniversary Edition by Marie Winn, © 1977, 1985, 2002 Marie Winn Miller. Used by permission of Viking Penguin, a division of Penguin Group (USA) Inc.

Chapter 7

Excerpts from *Four Arguments for the Elimination of Television* by Jerry Mander. © 1978 Jerry Mander. Reprinted by permission of HarperCollins Publishers.

Extract from *All Consuming Images* by Stuart Ewen, p 89. Copyright © 1988. Used by permission of Perseus Books Group.

Excerpts from *The Beauty Myth* by Naomi Wolf. Copyright © 1991 Naomi Wolf. Reprinted by permission of HarperCollins Publishers.

Index

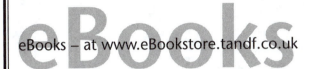

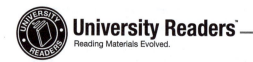

University Readers™
Reading Materials Evolved.

Introducing the

SOCIAL ISSUES
COLLECTION

A Routledge/University Readers Custom Library for Teaching

Customizing course material for innovative and excellent teaching in sociology has never been easier or more effective!

Choose from a collection of more than 300 readings from Routledge, Taylor & Francis, and other publishers to make a custom anthology that suits the needs of your social problems/ social inequality, and social issues courses.

All readings have been aptly chosen by academic editors and our authors and organized by topic and author.

Online tool makes it easy for busy instructors:

1. *Simply select your favorite Routledge and Taylor & Francis readings, and add any other required course material, including your own.*

2. *Choose the order of the readings, pick a binding, and customize a cover.*

3. *One click will post your materials for students to buy. They can purchase print or digital packs, and we ship direct to their door within two weeks of ordering!*

More information at www.socialissuescollection.com

Contact information: Call your Routledge sales rep, or
Becky Smith at University Readers, 800-200-3908 ext. 18, bsmith@universityreaders.com
Steve Rutter at Routledge, 207-434-2102, Steve.Rutter@taylorandfrancis.com.

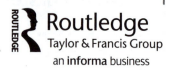

Routledge
Taylor & Francis Group
an **informa** business